LYMPHATIC DIET COOKBOOK

An Optimal Diet to Boost Immune System and Reduce Inflammation Including 170+ Nutritional Recipes to Maintain Healthy Living.

TABLE OF CONTENTS

CHAPTER 1: INTRODUCTION

The Lymphatic Diet is a gastronomic journey waiting to be discovered in the quiet nooks of wellness where the symphony of health meets the dance of nutrients. In a world where flavors and health collide and every meal is a step towards vitality. Allow the tantalizing tales of bright ingredients and nutritious recipes to unravel as you begin on this gastronomic voyage through the pages of our Lymphatic Diet cookbook painting a canvas of well-being that transcends the ordinary. It's time to appreciate not just the flavor but also the transformation. Welcome to a kitchen where every dish is a celebration of your body's harmony, a sensory symphony and a road map to a revitalized self.

UNDERSTANDING THE LYMPHATIC SYSTEM

The lymphatic system is a complicated network that parallels the circulatory system and serves as a silent conductor of health within our bodies. This system which consists of lymph nodes, veins and organs is the unsung hero of our immune defense and fluid homeostasis. Consider it a thorough waste disposal and filtration system that works hard to cleanse and purify. Lymph the fluid that runs through this complicated network, transports immune cells, nutrition and waste orchestrating a symphony of biological operations. Understanding the lymphatic system reveals its involvement in cleansing, immunological response and fluid balance. It is the body's protector gently ensuring balance and vitality.

BENEFITS OF A LYMPHATIC-FRIENDLY DIET

1. Immune System Support: A lymphatic-friendly diet includes critical nutrients that support the immune system assisting your body in fighting infections and illnesses.

2. Optimized Detoxification: By including meals that encourage lymphatic drainage such as fruits and vegetables you help your body remove toxins and enhance overall detoxification.

3. Improved Fluid Balance: A diet rich in hydrating foods and those known for their lymphatic advantages aids in the maintenance of adequate fluid balance lowering the risk of bloating and edema.

4. Reduced Inflammation: The anti-inflammatory qualities of particular foods in a lymphatic-friendly diet help to reduce inflammation and promote joint and tissue health.

5. Increased Energy: The nutrient-dense foods in this diet give prolonged energy, aiding in tiredness management and increasing vigor throughout the day.

6. Supporting the lymphatic system aids in the efficient evacuation of waste and excess fluids, which contributes to a healthy metabolism and may aid in weight management.

7. Hormone Balance: Some foods in a lymphatic-friendly diet may improve hormonal balance, promoting general well-being and potentially reducing symptoms associated with hormonal changes.

8. Radiant Skin: The lymphatic-friendly diet's cleansing tendency may be seen in your skin, producing a cleaner complexion and a healthy glow.

FOODS TO INCLUDE AND AVOID IN LYMPHATIC DIET

Lymphatic Diet Foods to Include:

1. Spinach, kale, and other leafy greens are high in chlorophyll and antioxidants, which aid in detoxifying.
2. Citrus Fruits: Oranges, lemons, and grapefruits are high in vitamin C, which supports immunological function and lymphatic health.
3. Berries: Blueberries, strawberries, and raspberries are high in antioxidants, which help fight inflammation and promote general health.
4. Turmeric, ginger, and garlic have anti-inflammatory effects, making them excellent additions to a lymphatic-friendly diet.
5. Cucumbers, watermelon, and celery all help with hydration, which is necessary for lymphatic fluid balance.
6. Lean Proteins: Include poultry, fish, and tofu to get the amino acids you need for cellular repair and immunological function.
7. Avocado, olive oil, and almonds are high in omega-3 fatty acids, which aid in anti-inflammatory activities.
8. Herbal Teas: Dandelion and ginger teas may aid in lymphatic movement and detoxifying.

Lymphatic Diet Foods to Avoid:

1. Processed Foods: Limit your consumption of processed and packaged foods, which frequently contain additives and preservatives.
2. Highly Refined Sugars: Limit your intake of sugary foods, as too much sugar might contribute to inflammation.

3. Saturated Fats: To maintain cardiovascular health, limit foods high in saturated fats, such as fried and fatty meats.

4. Excessive Dairy Consumption: While moderate dairy consumption is fine, excessive dairy consumption may contribute to congestion and inflammation in some people.

5. Alcohol consumption should be limited because it might dehydrate the body and potentially impede lymphatic function.

6. Sodium-Rich Foods: Because high sodium levels might cause water retention, it's best to limit your salt intake.

7. Processed Meats: Limit your consumption of processed meats such as sausages and hot dogs because they may include additives that are harmful to your overall health.

CHAPTER 2: FRIENDLY BREAKFAST OPTIONS

Green Smoothie Bowl:

Ingredients:

- 1 cup spinach leaves, washed
- 1/2 cucumber, peeled and sliced
- 1/2 avocado, peeled and pitted
- 1/2 banana, frozen
- 1/2 cup pineapple chunks, frozen
- 1/2 cup almond milk (or any plant-based milk)
- 1 tablespoon chia seeds
- Toppings: sliced kiwi, granola, shredded coconut and a drizzle of honey

Instructions:

1. In a blender, combine spinach, cucumber, avocado, banana, pineapple and almond milk.
2. Blend until smooth and creamy.
3. Pour the smoothie into a bowl.
4. Sprinkle chia seeds on top.
5. Arrange sliced kiwi, granola and shredded coconut as desired.
6. Drizzle honey over the toppings for added sweetness.
7. Enjoy your nutritious and delicious green smoothie bowl!

Citrus Salad:

Ingredients:

- 2 cups mixed greens (spinach, arugula and watercress)
- 1 grapefruit, peeled and segmented
- 1 orange, peeled and segmented
- 1/2 cup pomegranate seeds
- 1/4 cup pumpkin seeds

- 1 tablespoon fresh mint, chopped

Citrus Dressing:

- 2 tablespoons extra-virgin olive oil
- 1 tablespoon fresh lemon juice
- 1 teaspoon honey
- Salt and pepper to taste

Instructions:

1. In a large bowl, combine the mixed greens, grapefruit segments, orange segments, pomegranate seeds, pumpkin seeds and chopped mint.
2. In a small bowl, whisk together the olive oil, lemon juice, honey, salt and pepper to create the citrus dressing.
3. Drizzle the dressing over the salad and toss gently to coat evenly.
4. Allow the salad to marinate for a few minutes to enhance the flavors.
5. Serve the citrus salad chilled.

Avocado Toast with Poached Egg:

Ingredients:

- 1 ripe avocado
- 2 slices whole-grain bread, toasted
- 2 large eggs
- Salt and pepper to taste
- Red pepper flakes (optional)
- Chopped fresh chives for garnish

Instructions:

1. Toast the slices of whole-grain bread to your desired level of crispiness.
2. While the bread is toasting, cut the ripe avocado in half and remove the pit. Scoop the avocado flesh into a bowl and mash it with a fork. Add a pinch of salt and pepper and mix well.
3. Spread the mashed avocado evenly over the toasted bread slices.

4. In a saucepan, bring water to a gentle simmer. Add a splash of vinegar (optional) to help the eggs coagulate.

5. Crack one egg into a small bowl. Create a gentle whirlpool in the simmering water and carefully slide the egg into the center of the whirlpool. Poach the egg for about 3-4 minutes for a runny yolk or longer for a firmer yolk.

6. Use a slotted spoon to carefully lift the poached egg out of the water, allowing excess water to drain.

7. Place the poached egg on top of one of the avocado-covered toasts.

8. Repeat the poaching process with the second egg and place it on the second slice of toast.

9. Sprinkle with salt, pepper and red pepper flakes if desired. Garnish with chopped fresh chives.

10. Serve immediately and enjoy your delicious and nutritious avocado toast with poached egg!

Chia Seed Pudding:

Ingredients:

- 1/4 cup chia seeds
- 1 cup almond milk (or any preferred milk)
- 1 tablespoon maple syrup or honey (adjust to taste)
- 1/2 teaspoon vanilla extract
- Fresh fruits, nuts, or granola for toppings (optional)

Instructions:

1. In a bowl, combine the chia seeds, almond milk, maple syrup (or honey) and vanilla extract.

2. Whisk the ingredients together thoroughly to ensure the chia seeds are well distributed.

3. Let the mixture sit for a few minutes, then whisk again to prevent clumping.

4. Cover the bowl and refrigerate for at least 2 hours or overnight, allowing the chia seeds to absorb the liquid and create a pudding-like consistency.

5. After refrigeration, give the chia pudding a good stir.

6. Spoon the chia pudding into serving bowls or jars.

7. Top with fresh fruits, nuts or granola for added texture and flavor.

8. Drizzle with a bit more maple syrup if desired.

9. Serve chilled and enjoy a nutritious and satisfying chia seed pudding!

Greek Yogurt Parfait:

Ingredients:

- 1/4 cup chia seeds
- 1 cup almond milk (or any preferred milk)
- 1 tablespoon maple syrup or honey (adjust to taste)
- 1/2 teaspoon vanilla extract
- Fresh fruits, nuts or granola for toppings (optional)

Instructions:

1. In a bowl, combine the chia seeds, almond milk, maple syrup (or honey), and vanilla extract.

2. Whisk the ingredients together thoroughly to ensure the chia seeds are well distributed.

3. Let the mixture sit for a few minutes, then whisk again to prevent clumping.

4. Cover the bowl and refrigerate for at least 2 hours or overnight, allowing the chia seeds to absorb the liquid and create a pudding-like consistency.

5. After refrigeration, give the chia pudding a good stir.

6. Spoon the chia pudding into serving bowls or jars.

7. Top with fresh fruits, nuts or granola for added texture and flavor.

8. Drizzle with a bit more maple syrup if desired.

9. Serve chilled and enjoy a nutritious and satisfying chia seed pudding!

Oatmeal with Berries:

Ingredients:

- 1/2 cup old-fashioned oats
- 1 cup milk (dairy or plant-based)
- 1/2 teaspoon vanilla extract
- 1/2 cup mixed berries (strawberries, blueberries, raspberries)
- 1 tablespoon honey or maple syrup
- Chopped nuts (optional, for topping)

Instructions:

1. In a saucepan, combine the oats and milk. Bring to a gentle simmer over medium heat.
2. Stir in the vanilla extract and reduce the heat to low. Cook the oats, stirring occasionally, until they reach your desired consistency (usually 5-7 minutes).
3. While the oats are cooking, wash and prepare the mixed berries.
4. Once the oats are cooked, remove the saucepan from heat.
5. Spoon the oatmeal into a bowl and top with the mixed berries.
6. Drizzle honey or maple syrup over the berries for added sweetness.
7. Optional: Sprinkle chopped nuts (such as almonds or walnuts) on top for extra crunch and nutrition.
8. Serve warm and enjoy a delicious and wholesome oatmeal breakfast with a burst of berry goodness!

Quinoa Breakfast Bowl:

Ingredients:

- 1/2 cup quinoa, rinsed
- 1 cup water or milk (dairy or plant-based)
- 1 tablespoon chia seeds
- 1/2 teaspoon ground cinnamon
- 1 tablespoon honey or maple syrup

- Fresh fruits (such as sliced bananas, berries or kiwi)
- Nuts or seeds for topping (almonds, walnuts, or sunflower seeds)
- Greek yogurt or coconut yogurt (optional for topping)

Instructions:

1. Rinse the quinoa under cold water.
2. In a saucepan, combine quinoa and water (or milk). Bring to a boil, then reduce heat to low, cover and simmer for about 15 minutes or until the quinoa is cooked and the liquid is absorbed.
3. Stir in chia seeds, ground cinnamon, and honey (or maple syrup) into the cooked quinoa.
4. Remove the quinoa from heat, cover, and let it sit for 5 minutes to allow the chia seeds to absorb some liquid and thicken the mixture.
5. Fluff the quinoa with a fork and transfer it to a bowl.
6. Top the quinoa with fresh fruits of your choice.
7. Sprinkle nuts or seeds on top for added crunch and nutrition.
8. Optional: Add a dollop of Greek yogurt or coconut yogurt for creaminess.
9. Drizzle with a bit more honey or maple syrup if desired.
10. Serve warm and enjoy a wholesome and protein-packed quinoa breakfast bowl!

Smoked Salmon and Avocado Wrap:

Ingredients:

- 1 large whole-grain or spinach tortilla
- 2 ounces smoked salmon
- 1/2 ripe avocado, sliced
- 1 tablespoon cream cheese
- 1 teaspoon capers (optional)
- Fresh dill, chopped
- Baby spinach leaves
- Lemon wedges for serving

Instructions:

1. Lay the tortilla on a flat surface.
2. Spread cream cheese evenly over the tortilla, leaving a border around the edges.
3. Place a layer of baby spinach leaves on top of the cream cheese.
4. Arrange slices of smoked salmon over the spinach.
5. Add sliced avocado on top of the smoked salmon.
6. Sprinkle capers (if using) and chopped fresh dill over the avocado.
7. Gently fold in the sides of the tortilla and then roll it tightly from the bottom to create a wrap.
8. Slice the wrap in half diagonally for easier handling.
9. Serve with lemon wedges on the side for a burst of citrus flavor.
10. Enjoy your delicious and nutritious smoked salmon and avocado wrap!

Turmeric Scrambled Eggs:

Ingredients:

- 2 large eggs
- 1/4 teaspoon ground turmeric
- Salt and pepper to taste
- 1 tablespoon milk (optional)
- 1 tablespoon butter or oil for cooking
- Fresh parsley, chopped (for garnish, optional)

Instructions:

1. Crack the eggs into a bowl and whisk them until well combined.
2. Add ground turmeric, salt, and pepper to the whisked eggs. If you prefer creamier scrambled eggs, you can also add a tablespoon of milk at this stage.
3. Heat butter or oil in a non-stick skillet over medium-low heat.
4. Pour the egg mixture into the skillet.
5. Allow the eggs to sit undisturbed for a moment, then gently stir with a spatula, folding from the edges towards the center.

6. Continue stirring occasionally until the eggs are mostly set but still slightly runny.

7. Remove the skillet from heat as the residual heat will continue to cook the eggs to perfection.

8. Garnish with chopped fresh parsley if desired.

9. Serve immediately and enjoy your flavorful and turmeric-infused scrambled eggs!

Coconut Yogurt with Mango:

Ingredients:

- 1 cup coconut yogurt (store-bought or homemade)
- 1 ripe mango, peeled and diced
- 1 tablespoon honey or maple syrup (optional)
- 2 tablespoons shredded coconut
- Fresh mint leaves for garnish (optional)

Instructions:

1. Spoon coconut yogurt into a serving bowl.

2. Dice the ripe mango and arrange the mango cubes on top of the coconut yogurt.

3. If you prefer a sweeter taste, drizzle honey or maple syrup over the mango and yogurt.

4. Sprinkle shredded coconut evenly over the mixture for added texture and flavor.

5. Optional: Garnish with fresh mint leaves for a burst of freshness.

6. Serve immediately and enjoy your delicious and tropical coconut yogurt with mango!

Almond Butter Banana Pancakes:

Ingredients:

- 1 cup all-purpose flour or whole wheat flour
- 1 tablespoon baking powder
- 1/4 teaspoon salt
- 1 ripe banana, mashed

- 1 cup milk (dairy or plant-based)
- 2 tablespoons almond butter
- 1 tablespoon maple syrup or honey
- 1 teaspoon vanilla extract
- 1 egg
- Butter or oil for cooking

Instructions:

1. In a large bowl, whisk together the flour, baking powder and salt.
2. In a separate bowl, mash the ripe banana and add milk, almond butter, maple syrup (or honey) vanilla extract and the egg. Mix until well combined.
3. Pour the wet ingredients into the dry ingredients and stir until just combined. Do not overmix; a few lumps are okay.
4. Heat a griddle or non-stick skillet over medium heat and add a small amount of butter or oil.
5. Scoop 1/4 cup portions of batter onto the griddle for each pancake.
6. Cook until bubbles form on the surface, then flip and cook the other side until golden brown.
7. Repeat until all the batter is used.
8. Serve the pancakes warm with additional banana slices, a drizzle of almond butter and a touch of maple syrup.

Vegetable Omelet:

Ingredients:

- 3 large eggs
- 2 tablespoons milk
- Salt and pepper to taste
- 1 tablespoon olive oil or butter
- 1/4 cup bell peppers, diced
- 1/4 cup tomatoes, diced

- 1/4 cup red onion, finely chopped
- 1/4 cup spinach, chopped
- 1/4 cup mushrooms, sliced
- 1/4 cup shredded cheese (cheddar, feta or your choice)
- Fresh herbs (such as parsley or chives) for garnish (optional)

Instructions:

1. Crack the eggs into a bowl, add milk, salt and pepper and whisk until well combined.
2. Heat olive oil or butter in a non-stick skillet over medium heat.
3. Add bell peppers, tomatoes, red onion, spinach and mushrooms to the skillet. Saute until vegetables are tender but still slightly crisp.
4. Remove the vegetables from the skillet and set aside.
5. In the same skillet, add a bit more oil if needed and pour in the whisked eggs.
6. Allow the eggs to set slightly at the edges, then gently lift the edges with a spatula to let the uncooked eggs flow underneath.
7. Once the eggs are mostly set but still slightly runny on top, spread the sauteed vegetables over one-half of the omelet.
8. Sprinkle shredded cheese on top of the vegetables.
9. Carefully fold the other half of the omelet over the vegetables and cheese.
10. Cook for an additional minute or until the cheese is melted and the omelet is cooked through.
11. Slide the omelet onto a plate, garnish with fresh herbs if desired and serve immediately.

Quinoa Salad with Roasted Vegetables:

Ingredients:

- 1 cup quinoa
- 2 cups water or vegetable broth
- 2 cups mixed vegetables (e.g. bell peppers, cherry tomatoes, zucchini, red onion)
- 2 tablespoons olive oil
- Salt and pepper to taste
- 1/4 cup feta cheese (optional)
- Fresh herbs (e.g. parsley or basil) for garnish

For the Dressing:

- 3 tablespoons olive oil
- 2 tablespoons balsamic vinegar
- 1 teaspoon Dijon mustard
- Salt and pepper to taste

Instructions:

1. Preheat the oven: Preheat your oven to 400°F (200°C).
2. Prepare the Quinoa: Rinse the quinoa under cold water. In a saucepan, combine quinoa and water or vegetable broth. Bring to a boil, then reduce heat to low, cover and simmer for 15 minutes or until quinoa is cooked and water is absorbed. Fluff with a fork and let it cool.
3. Roast the Vegetables: Chop the mixed vegetables into bite-sized pieces. Toss them with olive oil, salt and pepper. Spread them on a baking sheet and roast in the preheated oven for about 20-25 minutes or until they are tender and slightly browned.
4. Make the Dressing: In a small bowl, whisk together olive oil, balsamic vinegar, Dijon mustard, salt and pepper.

5. Assemble the Salad: In a large bowl, combine the cooked quinoa, roasted vegetables and feta cheese if using. Pour the dressing over the salad and toss until everything is well coated.

6. Garnish and Serve: Sprinkle fresh herbs over the salad for a burst of flavor. Serve the quinoa salad either warm or at room temperature.

Grilled Chicken Wrap:

Ingredients:

- 1 pound boneless, skinless chicken breasts
- 2 tablespoons olive oil
- 1 teaspoon paprika
- 1 teaspoon garlic powder
- 1 teaspoon cumin
- Salt and pepper to taste
- 4 large tortillas or wraps
- 1 cup shredded lettuce
- 1 cup diced tomatoes
- 1/2 cup sliced red onions
- 1/2 cup shredded cheddar cheese
- Greek yogurt or your favorite dressing for drizzling

Instructions:

1. Prepare the Marinade: In a bowl, mix olive oil, paprika, garlic powder, cumin, salt and pepper to create a marinade.

2. Marinate the Chicken: Coat the chicken breasts with the marinade, ensuring they are well covered. Let it marinate for at least 30 minutes to allow the flavors to infuse.

3. Grill the Chicken: Preheat the grill or grill pan over medium-high heat. Grill the marinated chicken breasts for about 6-8 minutes per side or until fully cooked and internal temperature reaches 165°F (74°C).

4. Slice the Chicken: Once grilled, let the chicken rest for a few minutes, then slice it into thin strips.

5. Assemble the Wraps: Lay out the tortillas or wraps. Place a portion of sliced grilled chicken in the center of each wrap.

6. Add Toppings: Top the chicken with shredded lettuce, diced tomatoes, sliced red onions and shredded cheddar cheese.

7. Drizzle with Dressing: Drizzle Greek yogurt or your favorite dressing over the toppings for added flavor.

8. Wrap and Serve: Fold the sides of the tortilla over the filling and roll it up tightly into a wrap. Secure with toothpicks if needed. Repeat for the remaining wraps.

9. Serve: Serve the grilled chicken wraps immediately and enjoy a delicious and satisfying meal.

Mediterranean Chickpea Bowl:

Ingredients:

For the Chickpeas:

- 2 cans (15 oz each) chickpeas, drained and rinsed
- 2 tablespoons olive oil
- 1 teaspoon ground cumin
- 1 teaspoon smoked paprika
- Salt and pepper to taste

For the Bowl:

- 2 cups cooked quinoa or couscous
- 1 cup cherry tomatoes, halved
- 1 cucumber, diced
- 1/2 red onion, finely chopped
- 1/2 cup Kalamata olives, pitted and sliced
- 1/2 cup crumbled feta cheese (optional)
- Fresh parsley for garnish

For the Dressing:

- 1/4 cup extra-virgin olive oil
- 2 tablespoons red wine vinegar
- 1 clove garlic, minced
- 1 teaspoon dried oregano
- Salt and pepper to taste

Instructions:

1. Roast the Chickpeas: Preheat the oven to 400°F (200°C). In a bowl, toss chickpeas with olive oil, cumin, smoked paprika, salt and pepper. Spread them on a baking sheet and roast for 20-25 minutes or until they are crispy.

2. Prepare the Dressing: In a small bowl, whisk together olive oil, red wine vinegar, minced garlic, dried oregano, salt and pepper. Set aside.

3. Assemble the Bowl: In serving bowls, layer cooked quinoa or couscous, roasted chickpeas, cherry tomatoes, diced cucumber, chopped red onion, Kalamata olives and crumbled feta cheese if using.

4. Drizzle with Dressing: Drizzle the prepared dressing over the bowl ingredients.

5. Garnish and Serve: Garnish the Mediterranean Chickpea Bowl with fresh parsley. Serve immediately and enjoy the vibrant flavors of this nutritious bowl.

Salmon and Asparagus Foil Packets:

Ingredients:

- 4 salmon fillets
- 1 bunch of asparagus, trimmed
- 2 tablespoons olive oil
- 2 cloves garlic, minced
- 1 lemon, sliced
- Salt and pepper to taste
- Fresh dill for garnish (optional)
- 4 sheets of aluminum foil

Instructions:

1. Preheat the Oven: Preheat your oven to 400°F (200°C).

2. Prepare the Foil Packets: Place each salmon filet in the center of a sheet of aluminum foil. Arrange a portion of trimmed asparagus around each filet.

3. Season the Salmon and Asparagus: Drizzle olive oil over each salmon filet and asparagus bundle. Sprinkle minced garlic evenly over the top. Season with salt and pepper to taste.

4. Add Lemon Slices: Place lemon slices on top of each salmon filet. The lemon adds a burst of citrus flavor during cooking.

5. Fold and Seal the Packets: Fold the sides of the foil over the salmon and asparagus, creating a packet. Seal the edges tightly to prevent steam from escaping.

6. Bake in the Oven: Place the foil packets on a baking sheet and bake in the preheated oven for 15-20 minutes or until the salmon is cooked through and flakes easily with a fork.

7. Garnish and Serve: Carefully open the foil packets, being cautious of the hot steam. Garnish with fresh dill if desired. Serve the salmon and asparagus directly from the foil packets for a beautiful presentation.

8. Optional Grilling: Alternatively, you can cook these foil packets on a preheated grill for a smoky flavor. Grill for about 10-15 minutes.

Vegetarian Stir-Fry:

Ingredients:

- 1 cup broccoli florets
- 1 bell pepper, thinly sliced
- 1 carrot, julienned
- 1 zucchini, thinly sliced
- 1 cup snap peas, ends trimmed
- 1 cup tofu, cubed

- 3 tablespoons soy sauce
- 1 tablespoon sesame oil
- 1 tablespoon vegetable oil
- 2 cloves garlic, minced
- 1 teaspoon fresh ginger, grated
- 2 green onions, sliced
- Sesame seeds for garnish (optional)
- Cooked rice or noodles for serving

Instructions:

1. Prepare the Tofu: If using firm tofu, press it to remove excess water, then cut it into cubes.
2. Mix the Sauce: In a small bowl, whisk together soy sauce, sesame oil, minced garlic and grated ginger to create the stir-fry sauce.
3. Stir-Fry Vegetables: Heat vegetable oil in a wok or large skillet over medium-high heat. Add broccoli, bell pepper, carrot, zucchini and snap peas. Stir-fry for 4-5 minutes or until vegetables are crisp-tender.
4. Add Tofu: Push the vegetables to the side of the wok and add tofu cubes. Cook for an additional 2-3 minutes allowing the tofu to brown slightly.
5. Combine and Sauce: Combine the tofu with the vegetables in the wok. Pour the prepared sauce over the mixture and toss everything together until well-coated.
6. Finish Cooking: Continue stir-frying for an additional 2-3 minutes or until the tofu and vegetables are cooked to your liking.
7. Garnish and Serve: Remove the wok from heat. Garnish the stir-fry with sliced green onions and sesame seeds if desired. Serve the vegetarian stir-fry over cooked rice or noodles.

Quinoa-Stuffed Bell Peppers:

Ingredients:

- 4 large bell peppers, halved and seeds removed

- 1 cup quinoa, rinsed
- 2 cups vegetable broth or water
- 1 tablespoon olive oil
- 1 onion, finely chopped
- 2 cloves garlic, minced
- 1 zucchini, diced
- 1 tomato, diced
- 1 cup black beans, cooked or canned and drained
- 1 teaspoon ground cumin
- 1 teaspoon chili powder
- Salt and pepper to taste
- 1 cup shredded cheese (cheddar, mozzarella, or your choice)
- Fresh cilantro or parsley for garnish (optional)

Instructions:

1. Preheat the Oven: Preheat your oven to 375°F (190°C).
2. Cook Quinoa: In a saucepan, combine quinoa and vegetable broth or water. Bring to a boil, then reduce heat, cover and simmer for 15 minutes or until quinoa is cooked and liquid is absorbed. Fluff with a fork.
3. Prepare Bell Peppers: Cut the bell peppers in half lengthwise, removing seeds and membranes. Place the pepper halves in a baking dish.
4. Sauté Vegetables: In a large skillet, heat olive oil over medium heat. Add chopped onion, minced garlic and diced zucchini. Saute until the vegetables are softened.
5. Combine Ingredients: In a large bowl, combine the cooked quinoa, sauteed vegetables, diced tomato, black beans, ground cumin, chili powder, salt and pepper. Mix well.
6. Stuff Bell Peppers: Spoon the quinoa mixture into each bell pepper half, pressing down gently to pack the filling.
7. Add Cheese: Sprinkle shredded cheese over the top of each stuffed pepper.

8. Bake in the Oven: Cover the baking dish with aluminum foil and bake for 25-30 minutes. Then remove the foil and bake for an additional 10 minutes or until the cheese is melted and bubbly.

9. Garnish and Serve: Remove from the oven and let the stuffed peppers cool slightly. Garnish with fresh cilantro or parsley if desired. Serve and enjoy!

Caprese Salad with Balsamic Glaze:

Ingredients:

- 4 large tomatoes, sliced
- 1 pound fresh mozzarella cheese, sliced
- Fresh basil leaves
- Balsamic glaze
- Extra-virgin olive oil
- Salt and pepper to taste

Instructions:

1. Prepare Tomatoes and Mozzarella: Slice the tomatoes and fresh mozzarella cheese into even slices.

2. Arrange on a Plate: Alternately layer the tomato slices, mozzarella slices and fresh basil leaves on a serving plate.

3. Season with Salt and Pepper: Sprinkle salt and pepper over the arranged tomato and mozzarella slices to taste.

4. Drizzle with Olive Oil: Drizzle extra-virgin olive oil over the salad for added flavor. Use a good-quality olive oil for the best taste.

5. Balsamic Glaze: Drizzle balsamic glaze generously over the Caprese salad. The balsamic glaze adds a sweet and tangy touch.

6. Garnish: Optionally, garnish with additional fresh basil leaves for a burst of color and flavor.

7. Serve: Serve immediately as a refreshing and light appetizer or side dish.

Sweet Potato and Lentil Curry:

Ingredients:

- 1 cup dried red lentils, rinsed
- 2 large sweet potatoes, peeled and diced
- 1 onion, finely chopped
- 3 cloves garlic, minced
- 1-inch piece of ginger, grated
- 1 can (14 oz) diced tomatoes
- 1 can (14 oz) coconut milk
- 2 tablespoons curry powder
- 1 teaspoon ground cumin
- 1 teaspoon ground coriander
- 1/2 teaspoon turmeric
- 1/2 teaspoon cayenne pepper (adjust to taste)
- Salt and pepper to taste
- 2 tablespoons vegetable oil
- Fresh cilantro for garnish
- Cooked rice or naan for serving

Instructions:

1. Rinse Lentils: Rinse the red lentils under cold water until the water runs clear.
2. Saute Aromatics: In a large pot or Dutch oven, heat vegetable oil over medium heat. Add chopped onion and cook until softened. Add minced garlic and grated ginger and saute for an additional 1-2 minutes until fragrant.
3. Add Spices: Stir in curry powder, ground cumin, ground coriander, turmeric, cayenne pepper, salt, and pepper. Cook for 1-2 minutes to toast the spices.
4. Add Lentils and Vegetables: Add rinsed red lentils, diced sweet potatoes, diced tomatoes (with their juices) and coconut milk to the pot. Stir well to combine.
5. Simmer: Bring the mixture to a boil, then reduce the heat to low, cover and simmer for 20-25 minutes or until lentils and sweet potatoes are tender.

6. Adjust Seasoning: Taste and adjust the seasoning, adding more salt, pepper or cayenne pepper as needed.

7. Serve: Serve the sweet potato and lentil curry over cooked rice or with naan. Garnish with fresh cilantro.

Turkey and Avocado Lettuce Wraps:

Ingredients:

- 1 pound ground turkey
- 1 tablespoon olive oil
- 1 teaspoon cumin
- 1 teaspoon chili powder
- 1/2 teaspoon garlic powder
- Salt and pepper to taste
- 1 avocado, diced
- 1 cup cherry tomatoes, halved
- 1/2 red onion, finely chopped
- 1/4 cup fresh cilantro, chopped
- Juice of 1 lime
- Iceberg or butter lettuce leaves for wrapping

Instructions:

1. Cook Ground Turkey: In a large skillet, heat olive oil over medium heat. Add ground turkey and cook until browned, breaking it apart with a spoon as it cooks.

2. Season Turkey: Add cumin, chili powder, garlic powder, salt and pepper to the cooked turkey. Stir well to incorporate the spices. Cook for an additional 2-3 minutes until the turkey is well-seasoned.

3. Prepare Avocado Salsa: In a bowl, combine diced avocado, cherry tomatoes, red onion, cilantro and lime juice. Toss gently to mix.

4. Assemble Lettuce Wraps: Spoon the seasoned ground turkey into individual lettuce leaves, creating wraps. Top each with the avocado salsa.

5. Serve: Arrange the Turkey and Avocado Lettuce Wraps on a platter and serve immediately.

Shrimp and Quinoa Stir-Fry:

Ingredients:

- 1 cup quinoa, rinsed
- 2 cups water or vegetable broth
- 1 pound large shrimp, peeled and deveined
- 2 tablespoons soy sauce
- 1 tablespoon oyster sauce
- 1 tablespoon hoisin sauce
- 1 tablespoon sesame oil
- 1 tablespoon vegetable oil
- 3 cloves garlic, minced
- 1 tablespoon fresh ginger, grated
- 1 red bell pepper, thinly sliced
- 1 cup sugar snap peas, trimmed
- 2 green onions, sliced
- Sesame seeds for garnish (optional)

Instructions:

1. Prepare Quinoa: In a saucepan, combine quinoa and water or vegetable broth. Bring to a boil, then reduce heat, cover and simmer for 15 minutes or until quinoa is cooked. Fluff with a fork and set aside.
2. Marinate Shrimp: In a bowl, combine shrimp with soy sauce, oyster sauce and hoisin sauce. Let it marinate for about 10-15 minutes.
3. Stir-Fry Shrimp: Heat vegetable oil in a wok or large skillet over medium-high heat. Add minced garlic and grated ginger, stir-frying for 1 minute. Add marinated shrimp and cook until they turn pink and opaque. Remove the shrimp from the wok and set aside.

4. Stir-Fry Vegetables: In the same wok, add a bit more oil if needed. Stir-fry bell pepper and sugar snap peas until they are crisp-tender.

5. Combine and Finish: Add the cooked quinoa and cooked shrimp back into the wok. Drizzle with sesame oil and toss everything together until well combined and heated through.

6. Garnish and Serve: Garnish the Shrimp and Quinoa Stir-Fry with sliced green onions and sesame seeds if desired. Serve hot.

Chickpea and Spinach Stew:

Ingredients:

- 2 tablespoons olive oil
- 1 onion, finely chopped
- 3 cloves garlic, minced
- 1 teaspoon ground cumin
- 1 teaspoon ground coriander
- 1 teaspoon paprika
- 1/2 teaspoon cayenne pepper (adjust to taste)
- 1 can (15 oz) chickpeas, drained and rinsed
- 1 can (14 oz) diced tomatoes
- 4 cups fresh spinach leaves, washed and chopped
- 2 cups vegetable broth
- Salt and pepper to taste
- Fresh lemon wedges for serving
- Optional: Greek yogurt for garnish

Instructions:

1. Sauté Aromatics: In a large pot or Dutch oven, heat olive oil over medium heat. Add chopped onion and saute until softened. Add minced garlic and cook for an additional minute.

2. Add Spices: Stir in ground cumin, ground coriander, paprika and cayenne pepper. Cook for 1-2 minutes until the spices are fragrant.

3. Combine Chickpeas and Tomatoes: Add chickpeas and diced tomatoes (with their juices) to the pot. Stir well to combine.

4. Add Spinach: Pour in vegetable broth and add chopped spinach. Stir and bring the mixture to a simmer.

5. Simmer: Reduce heat to low, cover the pot and let the stew simmer for 15-20 minutes, allowing the flavors to meld and the spinach to wilt.

6. Season: Taste and season with salt and pepper as needed.

7. Serve: Ladle the Chickpea and Spinach Stew into bowls. Optionally, garnish with a dollop of Greek yogurt and serve with fresh lemon wedges on the side.

Vegetable and Hummus Wrap:

Ingredients:

- 4 large whole-grain or spinach tortillas
- 1 cup hummus (store-bought or homemade)
- 1 cup cherry tomatoes, halved
- 1 cucumber, thinly sliced
- 1 bell pepper (any color), thinly sliced
- 1 medium carrot, julienned or grated
- 1/2 red onion, thinly sliced
- 1 cup mixed salad greens (e.g., spinach, arugula, or lettuce)
- 1/4 cup feta cheese, crumbled (optional)
- 1 tablespoon balsamic glaze or your favorite dressing

Instructions:

1. Prepare the Hummus Wrap Base:
   - Lay out the tortillas on a clean surface.
   - Spread a generous layer of hummus over each tortilla, leaving a small border around the edges.

2. Add Vegetables:
   - o Arrange cherry tomatoes, cucumber slices, bell pepper strips, julienned carrot, red onion slices and mixed salad greens on the hummus-covered tortillas.
3. Optional Feta Cheese:
   - o If desired, sprinkle crumbled feta cheese over the vegetables for an extra layer of flavor.
4. Drizzle with Dressing:
   - o Drizzle balsamic glaze or your favorite dressing over the vegetables for added taste.
5. Wrap It Up:
   - o Fold the sides of the tortilla over the filling, then roll it up tightly from the bottom to create a wrap.
6. Slice and Serve:
   - o If preferred, slice the wraps in half diagonally. This makes them easier to handle and serve.
7. Serve and Enjoy:
   - o Serve the Vegetable and Hummus Wraps immediately or wrap them in parchment paper for a convenient and portable meal.

CHAPTER 4: NOURISHING DINNERS

Baked Lemon Garlic Salmon:

Ingredients:

- 4 salmon filets
- 2 tablespoons olive oil
- 2 cloves garlic, minced
- Zest of 1 lemon
- Juice of 1 lemon
- 1 teaspoon dried thyme
- Salt and pepper to taste
- Fresh parsley for garnish
- Lemon slices for serving

Instructions:

1. Preheat the Oven:
   - Preheat your oven to 400°F (200°C).
2. Prepare Salmon Filets:
   - Pat the salmon filets dry with paper towels.
   - Place the filets on a baking sheet lined with parchment paper or lightly greased.
3. Make Lemon Garlic Mixture:
   - In a small bowl, combine olive oil, minced garlic, lemon zest, lemon juice, dried thyme, salt and pepper. Mix well to create the lemon garlic marinade.
4. Marinate Salmon:
   - Brush the lemon garlic mixture over each salmon filet ensuring they are well-coated.
5. Bake the Salmon:

- Bake the salmon in the preheated oven for 12-15 minutes or until the salmon flakes easily with a fork. The cooking time may vary based on the thickness of your salmon filets.

6. Garnish and Serve:
   - Remove the salmon from the oven and garnish with fresh parsley.
   - Serve the Baked Lemon Garlic Salmon hot with additional lemon slices on the side.

Vegetarian Buddha Bowl:

Ingredients:
For the Base:
- 2 cups cooked quinoa or brown rice
- 1 cup chickpeas, cooked or canned and drained
- 2 cups mixed greens (spinach, kale, arugula, etc.)

Vegetable Toppings:
- 1 cup cherry tomatoes, halved
- 1 cucumber, sliced
- 1 avocado, sliced
- 1 cup shredded carrots
- 1 red bell pepper, sliced
- 1 cup broccoli florets, steamed

Protein and Extras:
- 1/2 cup hummus
- 1/4 cup feta cheese, crumbled (optional)
- Sunflower seeds or pumpkin seeds for garnish

For the Dressing:
- 3 tablespoons olive oil
- 2 tablespoons balsamic vinegar
- 1 tablespoon Dijon mustard
- 1 clove garlic, minced
- Salt and pepper to taste

Instructions:
1. Prepare the Base:
   - Divide the cooked quinoa or brown rice among the serving bowls.
   - Arrange a portion of chickpeas and mixed greens beside the grains.

2. Add Vegetable Toppings:
   - Arrange cherry tomatoes, cucumber slices, avocado slices, shredded carrots, red bell pepper slices and steamed broccoli florets in separate sections on top of the base.
3. Protein and Extras:
   - Add a dollop of hummus in the center of each bowl.
   - Sprinkle crumbled feta cheese on top if desired.
   - Garnish with sunflower seeds or pumpkin seeds.
4. Prepare the Dressing:
   - In a small bowl, whisk together olive oil, balsamic vinegar, Dijon mustard, minced garlic, salt and pepper.
5. Drizzle and Toss:
   - Drizzle the dressing over each Buddha Bowl.
   - Toss the ingredients together just before serving to coat everything in the flavorful dressing.
6. Serve and Enjoy:
   - Serve the Vegetarian Buddha Bowls immediately.

Grilled Chicken and Vegetable Skewers:

Ingredients:

- 1.5 lbs boneless, skinless chicken breasts, cut into bite-sized pieces
- 2 bell peppers (any color), cut into chunks
- 1 large red onion, cut into chunks
- 1 zucchini, sliced
- 1/4 cup olive oil
- 3 cloves garlic, minced
- 1 teaspoon dried oregano
- 1 teaspoon dried thyme
- 1 teaspoon paprika
- Salt and pepper to taste
- Wooden skewers, soaked in water for at least 30 minutes

Instructions:

1. In a bowl, mix olive oil, minced garlic, oregano, thyme, paprika, salt and pepper to create the marinade.

2. Place the chicken pieces in a resealable plastic bag or shallow dish. Pour half of the marinade over the chicken, ensuring all pieces are coated. Marinate in the refrigerator for at least 30 minutes.

3. Preheat the grill to medium-high heat.

4. Thread the marinated chicken, bell peppers, red onion and zucchini onto the soaked wooden skewers, alternating between the ingredients.

5. Brush the skewers with the remaining marinade.

6. Place the skewers on the preheated grill and cook for 10-15 minutes, turning occasionally, until the chicken is cooked through and vegetables are tender.

7. Serve the grilled chicken and vegetable skewers hot with your favorite dipping sauce or over a bed of rice.

Lentil and Vegetable Stew:

Ingredients:

- 1 cup dried green or brown lentils, rinsed and drained
- 1 onion, finely chopped
- 2 carrots, diced
- 2 celery stalks, chopped
- 3 cloves garlic, minced
- 1 can (14 oz) diced tomatoes
- 6 cups vegetable broth
- 1 teaspoon ground cumin
- 1 teaspoon ground coriander
- 1 teaspoon dried thyme
- 1 bay leaf
- Salt and pepper to taste
- 2 cups chopped kale or spinach

- 2 tablespoons olive oil
- Fresh parsley for garnish (optional)

Instructions:

1. In a large pot, heat olive oil over medium heat. Add chopped onions, carrots, and celery. Saute until vegetables are softened, about 5 minutes.
2. Add minced garlic, ground cumin, ground coriander, dried thyme and cook for an additional 2 minutes until fragrant.
3. Pour in the vegetable broth, add lentils, diced tomatoes (with their juice) and bay leaf. Season with salt and pepper. Bring the mixture to a boil, then reduce the heat to low, cover and simmer for 25-30 minutes or until lentils are tender.
4. Add chopped kale or spinach to the pot and stir until wilted.
5. Adjust the seasoning if needed. Remove the bay leaf.
6. Serve the lentil and vegetable stew hot, garnished with fresh parsley if desired.

Zucchini Noodles with Pesto and Cherry Tomatoes:

Ingredients:

- 4 medium-sized zucchini, spiralized into noodles
- 1 cup cherry tomatoes, halved
- 1/2 cup grated Parmesan cheese
- 1/2 cup pine nuts, toasted
- 2 cups fresh basil leaves
- 2 cloves garlic
- 1/2 cup extra-virgin olive oil
- Salt and pepper to taste
- Red pepper flakes (optional, for added spice)

Instructions:

1. Prepare Zucchini Noodles:
   - Spiralize the zucchini into noodles using a spiralizer. Set aside.
2. Make Pesto:

- o In a food processor, combine basil, garlic, pine nuts and Parmesan cheese.
  - o Pulse until ingredients are finely chopped.
  - o With the food processor running, gradually pour in the olive oil until the pesto reaches a smooth consistency. Season with salt and pepper to taste.
3. Combine Zucchini Noodles and Pesto:
  - o In a large skillet, heat a bit of olive oil over medium heat.
  - o Add zucchini noodles and saute for 2-3 minutes until just tender but still crisp.
4. Mix in Pesto and Tomatoes:
  - o Add the pesto to the zucchini noodles, tossing to coat evenly.
  - o Stir in the halved cherry tomatoes and cook for an additional 2 minutes until the tomatoes are slightly softened.
5. Serve:
  - o Remove from heat and garnish with extra Parmesan cheese and toasted pine nuts.
  - o Optionally, sprinkle red pepper flakes for some heat.
6. Enjoy:
  - o Serve immediately.

Turkey and Vegetable Stir-Fry:

Ingredients:

- 1 lb ground turkey
- 2 tablespoons soy sauce
- 1 tablespoon oyster sauce
- 1 tablespoon hoisin sauce
- 2 tablespoons vegetable oil
- 1 onion, thinly sliced
- 1 bell pepper, thinly sliced (any color)
- 1 zucchini, thinly sliced

- 1 cup broccoli florets
- 2 carrots, julienned
- 3 cloves garlic, minced
- 1 tablespoon fresh ginger, grated
- Green onions, chopped for garnish
- Sesame seeds for garnish (optional)
- Cooked rice or noodles for serving

Instructions:

1. Prepare the Sauce:
   - In a small bowl, mix together soy sauce, oyster sauce and hoisin sauce. Set aside.
2. Cook Ground Turkey:
   - In a wok or large skillet, heat 1 tablespoon of vegetable oil over medium-high heat.
   - Add ground turkey and cook until browned. Remove any excess fat.
3. Stir-Fry Vegetables:
   - Push the turkey to one side of the wok. Add another tablespoon of oil to the empty side.
   - Add sliced onion, bell pepper, zucchini, broccoli and julienned carrots. Stir-fry the vegetables until they are tender-crisp.
4. Combine Turkey and Vegetables:
   - Mix the cooked turkey with the stir-fried vegetables in the wok.
5. Add Garlic and Ginger:
   - Create a well in the center of the wok. Add minced garlic and grated ginger. Stir briefly until fragrant.
6. Combine Sauce and Finish:
   - Pour the sauce over the turkey and vegetable mixture. Stir everything together until well-coated and heated through.
7. Serve:

- Serve the turkey and vegetable stir-fry over cooked rice or noodles.

Eggplant and Chickpea Curry:

Ingredients:

- 1 large eggplant, diced
- 1 can (15 oz) chickpeas, drained and rinsed
- 1 onion, finely chopped
- 3 cloves garlic, minced
- 1 tablespoon ginger, grated
- 1 can (14 oz) diced tomatoes
- 1 can (14 oz) coconut milk
- 2 tablespoons curry powder
- 1 teaspoon ground cumin
- 1 teaspoon ground coriander
- 1/2 teaspoon turmeric
- 1/2 teaspoon cayenne pepper (adjust to taste)
- Salt and pepper to taste
- 2 tablespoons vegetable oil
- Fresh cilantro for garnish
- Cooked rice for serving

Instructions:

1. Prepare Eggplant:
   - Sprinkle diced eggplant with salt and let it sit for 15-20 minutes. Rinse and pat dry to reduce bitterness.
2. Saute Onion, Garlic and Ginger:
   - In a large pot, heat vegetable oil over medium heat. Add chopped onion and saute until softened.
   - Add minced garlic and grated ginger, cooking for an additional minute until fragrant.

3. Add Spices:
   - o Stir in curry powder, ground cumin, ground coriander, turmeric, cayenne pepper, salt and pepper. Cook for 1-2 minutes to toast the spices.
4. Cook Eggplant and Chickpeas:
   - o Add diced eggplant and chickpeas to the pot. Stir to coat them with the spice mixture.
5. Pour in Tomatoes and Coconut Milk:
   - o Pour in diced tomatoes (with their juice) and coconut milk. Stir to combine.
6. Simmer:
   - o Bring the curry to a simmer. Cover and let it cook for 20-25 minutes or until the eggplant is tender.
7. Adjust Seasoning and Serve:
   - o Taste and adjust the seasoning if needed. If you prefer more heat, add additional cayenne pepper.
   - o Serve the eggplant and chickpea curry over cooked rice.
8. Garnish:
   - o Garnish with fresh cilantro before serving.

Cauliflower Rice Bowl with Black Beans:

Ingredients:

- 1 medium-sized cauliflower, riced (use a food processor or box grater)
- 1 can (15 oz) black beans, drained and rinsed
- 1 cup corn kernels (fresh or frozen)
- 1 bell pepper, diced
- 1 small red onion, finely chopped
- 2 cloves garlic, minced
- 1 teaspoon ground cumin
- 1 teaspoon chili powder
- 1/2 teaspoon smoked paprika

- Salt and pepper to taste
- 2 tablespoons olive oil
- Juice of 1 lime
- Avocado slices for garnish
- Fresh cilantro for garnish
- Optional toppings: salsa, Greek yogurt, shredded cheese

Instructions:

1. Prepare Cauliflower Rice:
   - Rice the cauliflower using a food processor or box grater. Set aside.
2. Sauté Vegetables:
   - In a large skillet, heat olive oil over medium heat. Add diced bell pepper, chopped red onion and minced garlic. Saute until the vegetables are softened.
3. Add Black Beans and Corn:
   - Stir in black beans and corn kernels. Cook for an additional 2-3 minutes until heated through.
4. Season the Mixture:
   - Sprinkle ground cumin, chili powder, smoked paprika, salt and pepper over the vegetable and bean mixture. Stir to evenly coat.
5. Add Cauliflower Rice:
   - Add the riced cauliflower to the skillet. Stir well to combine with the vegetable and bean mixture.
6. Cook Until Tender:
   - Cook the cauliflower rice mixture for 5-7 minutes, stirring occasionally, until the cauliflower is tender but not mushy.
7. Finish and Serve:
   - Squeeze the lime juice over the cauliflower rice. Stir to combine.
   - Serve the cauliflower rice and black bean mixture in bowls.

- Garnish with avocado slices, fresh cilantro and any additional toppings you prefer.

Shrimp and Quinoa Salad:

Ingredients:

- 1 cup quinoa, rinsed and drained
- 1 pound large shrimp, peeled and deveined
- 1 tablespoon olive oil
- 1 teaspoon smoked paprika
- 1 teaspoon garlic powder
- Salt and pepper to taste
- 1 cucumber, diced
- 1 cup cherry tomatoes, halved
- 1/2 red onion, finely chopped
- 1/4 cup fresh parsley, chopped
- 1/4 cup feta cheese, crumbled (optional)

For the Dressing:

- 3 tablespoons extra-virgin olive oil
- 2 tablespoons red wine vinegar
- 1 teaspoon Dijon mustard
- Salt and pepper to taste

Instructions:

1. Cook Quinoa:
   - In a medium saucepan, combine quinoa with 2 cups of water. Bring to a boil, then reduce heat, cover and simmer for 15 minutes or until quinoa is cooked and water is absorbed. Fluff with a fork and let it cool.
2. Prepare Shrimp:

    o In a bowl, toss shrimp with olive oil, smoked paprika, garlic powder, salt and pepper. Heat a skillet over medium-high heat and cook the shrimp for 2-3 minutes per side until opaque and cooked through.

3. Make Dressing:
   - In a small bowl, whisk together olive oil, red wine vinegar, Dijon mustard, salt and pepper to create the dressing.

4. Assemble Salad:
   - In a large bowl, combine cooked quinoa, cooked shrimp, diced cucumber, cherry tomatoes, chopped red onion and fresh parsley.

5. Add Dressing:
   - Pour the dressing over the salad and toss to coat everything evenly.

6. Garnish:
   - Optionally, sprinkle crumbled feta cheese over the top for added flavor.

7. Chill and Serve:
   - Refrigerate the shrimp and quinoa salad for at least 30 minutes to allow the flavors to meld.
   - Serve chilled and enjoy a refreshing and protein-packed salad!

Stuffed Bell Peppers with Turkey and Quinoa:

Ingredients:

- 4 large bell peppers, halved and seeds removed
- 1 cup quinoa, rinsed
- 2 cups water or vegetable broth
- 1 tablespoon olive oil
- 1 onion, finely chopped
- 2 cloves garlic, minced
- 1 pound ground turkey
- 1 can (14 oz) diced tomatoes, drained
- 1 teaspoon ground cumin

- 1 teaspoon smoked paprika
- Salt and pepper to taste
- 1 cup black beans, drained and rinsed
- 1 cup corn kernels (fresh or frozen)
- 1 cup shredded cheese (cheddar, Monterey Jack, or a blend)
- Fresh cilantro for garnish (optional)

Instructions:

1. Preheat the Oven:
   - Preheat the oven to 375°F (190°C).
2. Cook Quinoa:
   - In a medium saucepan, combine quinoa and water or vegetable broth. Bring to a boil, then reduce heat, cover and simmer for 15 minutes or until quinoa is cooked. Fluff with a fork and set aside.
3. Prepare Bell Peppers:
   - Cut the bell peppers in half lengthwise and remove seeds. Place them in a baking dish.
4. Sauté Onion and Garlic:
   - In a large skillet, heat olive oil over medium heat. Add chopped onion and cook until softened. Add minced garlic and cook for an additional minute.
5. Cook Turkey:
   - Add ground turkey to the skillet and cook until browned. Drain excess fat.
6. Season and Add Vegetables:
   - Stir in diced tomatoes, ground cumin, smoked paprika, salt and pepper. Add black beans and corn. Mix well.
7. Combine Quinoa and Turkey Mixture:
   - Add the cooked quinoa to the turkey and vegetable mixture. Mix thoroughly.
8. Stuff Bell Peppers:
   - Spoon the turkey and quinoa mixture into each bell pepper half, pressing down gently.
9. Top with Cheese:
   - Sprinkle shredded cheese over the stuffed peppers.
10. Bake:
    - Cover the baking dish with foil and bake in the preheated oven for 25-30 minutes or until the peppers are tender.

11. Garnish and Serve:
    o Garnish with fresh cilantro if desired. Serve the stuffed bell peppers hot.

Broccoli and Tofu Stir-Fry:

Ingredients:

- 1 block (14 oz) extra-firm tofu, pressed and cubed
- 3 cups broccoli florets
- 1 red bell pepper, thinly sliced
- 1 carrot, julienned
- 3 cloves garlic, minced
- 1 tablespoon fresh ginger, grated
- 1/4 cup soy sauce
- 2 tablespoons hoisin sauce
- 1 tablespoon rice vinegar
- 1 tablespoon sesame oil
- 2 tablespoons vegetable oil
- 1 tablespoon cornstarch mixed with 2 tablespoons water (optional, for thickening)
- Cooked brown rice or noodles for serving
- Sesame seeds and sliced green onions for garnish

Instructions:

1. Prepare Tofu:
    o Press the tofu to remove excess water, then cut it into cubes.
2. Stir-Fry Tofu:
    o In a large wok or skillet, heat vegetable oil over medium-high heat. Add tofu cubes and stir-fry until golden brown on all sides. Remove tofu from the pan and set aside.
3. Cook Vegetables:
    o In the same pan, add a bit more oil if needed. Stir in minced garlic and grated ginger. Cook for about 1 minute until fragrant.
    o Add broccoli, red bell pepper, and julienned carrot. Stir-fry for 4-5 minutes until the vegetables are crisp-tender.
4. Combine Tofu and Vegetables:

○ Return the cooked tofu to the pan with the vegetables. Mix well.

5. Prepare Sauce:
   ○ In a small bowl, whisk together soy sauce, hoisin sauce, rice vinegar and sesame oil.
6. Add Sauce to Stir-Fry:
   ○ Pour the sauce over the tofu and vegetables. Stir to coat everything evenly.
7. Thicken Sauce (Optional):
   ○ If desired, mix cornstarch with water to create a slurry. Add it to the stir-fry to thicken the sauce. Stir well.
8. Serve:
   ○ Serve the broccoli and tofu stir-fry over cooked brown rice or noodles.
9. Garnish:
   ○ Garnish with sesame seeds and sliced green onions.

Mushroom and Spinach Stuffed Chicken Breast:

Ingredients:

- 4 boneless, skinless chicken breasts
- 1 cup baby spinach, chopped
- 1 cup mushrooms, finely chopped
- 1/2 cup feta cheese, crumbled
- 2 cloves garlic, minced
- 1 tablespoon olive oil
- 1 teaspoon dried oregano
- 1 teaspoon dried thyme
- Salt and pepper to taste
- 2 tablespoons butter, melted
- Toothpicks for securing

Instructions:

1. Preheat Oven:
   ○ Preheat the oven to 400°F (200°C).
2. Prepare Mushroom and Spinach Filling:

- o In a skillet, heat olive oil over medium heat. Add minced garlic and sauté for 1 minute.
  - o Add chopped mushrooms and cook until they release their moisture and become golden brown.
  - o Stir in chopped spinach and cook until wilted. Remove from heat and let it cool.
3. Make the Stuffing:
  - o In a bowl, combine the mushroom and spinach mixture with crumbled feta cheese, dried oregano, dried thyme, salt and pepper.
4. Prepare Chicken Breasts:
  - o Lay the chicken breasts flat and cut a pocket horizontally into each, being careful not to cut through the other side.
5. Stuff Chicken Breasts:
  - o Stuff each chicken breast pocket with the mushroom and spinach filling. Use toothpicks to secure the edges and keep the filling in place.
6. Season and Arrange:
  - o Place the stuffed chicken breasts in a baking dish. Brush melted butter over the top of each breast.
  - o Season the outside of the chicken breasts with additional salt, pepper, oregano and thyme.
7. Bake:
  - o Bake in the preheated oven for 25-30 minutes or until the chicken is cooked through and reaches an internal temperature of 165°F (74°C).
8. Serve:
  - o Remove toothpicks before serving.
  - o Serve the mushroom and spinach stuffed chicken breasts with your favorite side dishes.

Mixed Berry Smoothie:

Ingredients:

- 1 cup mixed berries (strawberries, blueberries, raspberries, blackberries)
- 1 ripe banana, peeled
- 1/2 cup plain Greek yogurt
- 1/2 cup almond milk (or any milk of your choice)
- 1 tablespoon honey or maple syrup (optional depending on sweetness preference)
- Ice cubes (optional)
- Fresh mint leaves for garnish (optional)

Instructions:

1. Prepare the Berries:
   - If using fresh berries, wash them thoroughly. If using frozen berries, no need to thaw.
2. Combine Ingredients:
   - In a blender, combine mixed berries, peeled banana, Greek yogurt, almond milk and honey (if desired).
3. Blend Until Smooth:
   - Blend all the ingredients until smooth and creamy. If the smoothie is too thick, you can add more almond milk to reach your preferred consistency.
4. Adjust Sweetness:
   - Taste the smoothie and add more honey or sweetener if needed.
5. Add Ice Cubes (Optional):
   - If you prefer a colder smoothie, add a handful of ice cubes and blend again until the ice is crushed and the smoothie is chilled.
6. Serve:
   - Pour the mixed berry smoothie into glasses.

7. Garnish (Optional):
    o Garnish with fresh mint leaves for a burst of freshness.
8. Enjoy:
    o Serve immediately and enjoy your refreshing mixed berry smoothie!

Vegetable Sticks with Hummus:

Ingredients:

- Assorted vegetables (carrots, cucumber, bell peppers, celery, cherry tomatoes, etc.)
- Hummus (store-bought or homemade)
- Olive oil (optional for drizzling)
- Fresh herbs (parsley, cilantro) for garnish (optional)
- Salt and pepper to taste

Instructions:

1. Prepare Vegetables:
    o Wash and peel (if necessary) the vegetables. Cut them into sticks or bite-sized pieces.
2. Arrange on a Platter:
    o Arrange the vegetable sticks on a serving platter. You can organize them in a colorful and appealing way.
3. Serve with Hummus:
    o Place a bowl of hummus in the center of the platter or distribute small individual portions.
4. Drizzle with Olive Oil (Optional):
    o Optionally, drizzle a bit of olive oil over the hummus for extra flavor.
5. Season with Salt and Pepper:
    o Sprinkle a pinch of salt and pepper over the vegetable sticks. Adjust according to taste.
6. Garnish (Optional):
    o Garnish with fresh herbs like parsley or cilantro for a touch of freshness.

7. Serve:
   - Serve the vegetable sticks with hummus as a healthy and delicious snack

Greek Yogurt with Almonds and Honey:

Ingredients:

- 1 cup Greek yogurt
- 2 tablespoons almonds, chopped
- 1 tablespoon honey (adjust to taste)
- Fresh berries (optional for garnish)
- Mint leaves (optional for garnish)

Instructions:

1. Spoon Greek Yogurt:
   - Spoon the Greek yogurt into a serving bowl or individual bowls.
2. Add Chopped Almonds:
   - Sprinkle the chopped almonds over the Greek yogurt.
3. Drizzle with Honey:
   - Drizzle honey over the yogurt and almonds. Adjust the amount according to your desired level of sweetness.
4. Garnish (Optional):
   - If desired, garnish with fresh berries like strawberries or blueberries and mint leaves for added freshness.
5. Serve:
   - Serve immediately.

Chia Seed Pudding with Berries:

Ingredients:

- 1/4 cup chia seeds
- 1 cup milk (almond milk, coconut milk, or any milk of your choice)
- 1 tablespoon maple syrup or honey (adjust to taste)

- 1/2 teaspoon vanilla extract
- Mixed berries (strawberries, blueberries, raspberries) for topping
- Nuts or granola for added crunch (optional)

Instructions:

1. Mix Chia Seeds and Milk:
   - In a bowl or jar, combine chia seeds and milk. Stir well to ensure the chia seeds are evenly distributed.
2. Add Sweetener and Vanilla:
   - Add maple syrup or honey and vanilla extract to the chia seed mixture. Stir again to combine.
3. Refrigerate Overnight:
   - Cover the bowl or jar and refrigerate the chia seed mixture for at least 4 hours or ideally, overnight. This allows the chia seeds to absorb the liquid and create a pudding-like consistency.
4. Stir Before Serving:
   - Before serving, give the chia seed pudding a good stir to break up any clumps and ensure a smooth texture.
5. Top with Berries:
   - Spoon the chia seed pudding into serving bowls or glasses. Top with mixed berries.
6. Add Crunchy Toppings (Optional):
   - For added texture, sprinkle nuts or granola on top of the berries.
7. Serve and Enjoy:
   - Serve the chia seed pudding with berries immediately and enjoy.

Sliced Apple with Almond Butter:

Ingredients:

- 1 apple, sliced
- 2 tablespoons almond butter

- Optional toppings: sliced almonds, chia seeds, cinnamon

Instructions:

1. Slice the Apple:

   o Wash and core the apple. Slice it into thin, even slices.

2. Spread Almond Butter:

   o Spread almond butter over each apple slice. You can use a knife or simply dip the apple slices directly into the almond butter.

3. Optional Toppings:

   o Optionally, sprinkle sliced almonds, chia seeds or a pinch of cinnamon over the almond butter.

4. Arrange and Serve:

   o Arrange the apple slices on a plate or serve them in a stack.

5. Enjoy:

   o Enjoy this simple and nutritious snack of sliced apple with almond butter!

Roasted Chickpeas:

Ingredients:

- 1 can (15 oz) chickpeas (garbanzo beans), drained and rinsed
- 1 tablespoon olive oil
- 1 teaspoon ground cumin
- 1 teaspoon smoked paprika
- 1/2 teaspoon garlic powder
- 1/2 teaspoon onion powder
- 1/2 teaspoon chili powder (adjust to taste)
- Salt to taste

Instructions:

1. Preheat Oven:

   o Preheat your oven to 400°F (200°C).

2. Prepare Chickpeas:

o Drain and rinse the chickpeas. Pat them dry using a paper towel to remove excess moisture.

3. Season Chickpeas:
   o In a bowl, toss the chickpeas with olive oil, ground cumin, smoked paprika, garlic powder, onion powder, chili powder and salt. Ensure that the chickpeas are evenly coated.

4. Spread on Baking Sheet:
   o Spread the seasoned chickpeas in a single layer on a baking sheet. Make sure they are not crowded to allow for even roasting.

5. Roast in the Oven:
   o Roast the chickpeas in the preheated oven for 20-25 minutes or until they become golden brown and crispy. Shake the pan or stir the chickpeas halfway through the cooking time for even roasting.

6. Cool and Serve:
   o Remove the roasted chickpeas from the oven and let them cool for a few minutes.

Kale Chips:

Ingredients:

- 1 bunch of kale
- 1-2 tablespoons olive oil
- Salt, to taste
- Optional: Seasonings like garlic powder, paprika or nutritional yeast

Instructions:

1. Preheat your oven to 350°F (175°C).
2. Wash the kale leaves thoroughly and pat them dry with a paper towel.
3. Remove the tough stems from the kale and tear the leaves into bite-sized pieces.
4. Place the torn kale in a large bowl and drizzle olive oil over it. Massage the oil into the leaves, ensuring they are evenly coated.

5. Spread the kale in a single layer on a baking sheet. Make sure not to overcrowd the leaves to ensure crispiness.

6. Sprinkle salt over the kale, and if desired, add your chosen seasonings for extra flavor.

7. Bake in the preheated oven for 10-15 minutes, or until the edges of the kale are browned and crispy. Keep an eye on them to prevent burning.

8. Remove from the oven and let the kale chips cool for a few minutes before serving.

Edamame Pods:

Ingredients:

- 1 pound (about 450g) fresh or frozen edamame pods
- 1-2 tablespoons sea salt (for boiling)
- Optional: Additional sea salt or soy sauce for seasoning

Instructions:

1. If using frozen edamame, thaw them according to the package instructions.

2. In a large pot, bring water to a boil. Add 1-2 tablespoons of sea salt to the boiling water.

3. Add the edamame pods to the boiling water. Cook for about 4-5 minutes or until the pods are tender.

4. Drain the edamame pods and transfer them to a bowl.

5. If desired, sprinkle additional sea salt or drizzle soy sauce over the edamame for added flavor. Toss to coat evenly.

6. Serve the edamame pods warm. To eat, simply pop the beans out of the pods into your mouth.

Trail Mix with Nuts and Dried Berries:

Ingredients:

- 1 cup almonds

- 1 cup walnuts
- 1 cup cashews
- 1 cup dried cranberries
- 1 cup dried blueberries
- 1 cup pumpkin seeds
- 1 cup dark chocolate chips or chunks (optional)
- 1/2 teaspoon sea salt (optional)

Instructions:

1. In a large mixing bowl, combine almonds, walnuts, cashews, dried cranberries, dried blueberries and pumpkin seeds.
2. If desired, add dark chocolate chips or chunks to the mix for a sweet touch.
3. If you like a hint of saltiness, sprinkle sea salt over the mixture. Toss everything together until well combined.
4. Store the trail mix in an airtight container to keep it fresh.
5. Shake or stir the mix before serving to ensure an even distribution of ingredients.
6. Portion out the trail mix into snack-sized bags or containers for a convenient and healthy on-the-go snack.

Cottage Cheese with Pineapple:

Ingredients:

- 1 cup cottage cheese
- 1 cup fresh pineapple chunks or canned pineapple tidbits (drained)
- 1 tablespoon honey (optional)
- Mint leaves for garnish (optional)

Instructions:

1. In a bowl, combine the cottage cheese and fresh pineapple chunks or drained canned pineapple tidbits.
2. Gently stir the mixture to evenly distribute the pineapple throughout the cottage cheese.

3. If you prefer a touch of sweetness, drizzle honey over the cottage cheese and pineapple mixture. Stir again to incorporate.

4. Garnish with mint leaves for a refreshing touch (optional).

5. Serve immediately and enjoy this simple and delicious cottage cheese with pineapple snack.

Turmeric Roasted Cashews:

Ingredients:

- 2 cups raw cashews
- 1 tablespoon olive oil
- 1 teaspoon ground turmeric
- 1/2 teaspoon ground cumin
- 1/2 teaspoon paprika
- 1/2 teaspoon garlic powder
- 1/2 teaspoon sea salt, or to taste

Instructions:

1. Preheat your oven to 325°F (163°C) and line a baking sheet with parchment paper.

2. In a large bowl, combine raw cashews with olive oil, ground turmeric, ground cumin, paprika, garlic powder and sea salt.

3. Toss the cashews until they are evenly coated with the spice mixture.

4. Spread the seasoned cashews in a single layer on the prepared baking sheet.

5. Roast in the preheated oven for 15-20 minutes or until the cashews are golden brown and fragrant. Stir halfway through the roasting time for even cooking.

6. Remove from the oven and let the turmeric roasted cashews cool completely before serving.

7. Store in an airtight container to maintain freshness.

Rice Cake with Avocado and Tomato:

Ingredients:

- 1 rice cake
- 1/2 ripe avocado, sliced
- 1 small tomato, sliced
- Salt and pepper to taste
- Optional: Red pepper flakes or your favorite seasoning

Instructions:

1. Place the rice cake on a plate or a flat surface.
2. Spread the sliced avocado evenly over the rice cake.
3. Arrange the tomato slices on top of the avocado.
4. Sprinkle salt and pepper to taste over the avocado and tomato.
5. Optionally, add a pinch of red pepper flakes or your preferred seasoning for an extra kick.
6. Serve immediately.

Sliced Cucumber with Tzatziki:

Ingredients:

- 1 cucumber, thinly sliced
- 1 cup Greek yogurt
- 1/2 cucumber, finely diced
- 2 tablespoons fresh dill, chopped
- 1 clove garlic, minced
- 1 tablespoon extra-virgin olive oil
- 1 tablespoon lemon juice
- Salt and pepper to taste

Instructions:

1. In a bowl, combine Greek yogurt, finely diced cucumber, chopped fresh dill, minced garlic, extra-virgin olive oil and lemon juice.
2. Mix the ingredients well until the tzatziki sauce is smooth and well-blended.
3. Arrange the thinly sliced cucumber on a serving platter.

4. Spoon the tzatziki sauce over the cucumber slices, ensuring an even distribution.

5. Sprinkle salt and pepper to taste over the cucumber and tzatziki.

6. Optionally, garnish with additional dill or a drizzle of olive oil.

7. Serve immediately and enjoy this refreshing and flavorful sliced cucumber with tzatziki.

Seaweed Snacks:

Ingredients:

- 1 package (about 10 sheets) roasted seaweed/nori sheets
- 1 tablespoon sesame oil
- 1 teaspoon soy sauce
- 1/2 teaspoon toasted sesame seeds
- Optional: Pinch of salt or seasoning of your choice

Instructions:

1. Lay the seaweed sheets flat on a clean surface.

2. In a small bowl, mix sesame oil and soy sauce.

3. Using a brush or your fingers, lightly brush each seaweed sheet with the sesame oil and soy sauce mixture.

4. Sprinkle toasted sesame seeds evenly over the seaweed sheets.

5. Optionally, add a pinch of salt or your preferred seasoning for added flavor.

6. Gently press the sesame seeds and seasoning onto the seaweed to help them adhere.

7. Cut or tear the seaweed sheets into bite-sized pieces.

8. Allow the seaweed snacks to sit for a few minutes to let the flavors meld.

9. Serve and enjoy these savory and crunchy homemade seaweed snacks.

Hard-Boiled Eggs with Paprika:

Ingredients:

- 4 large eggs

- Water for boiling
- 1/2 teaspoon paprika
- Salt and pepper, to taste
- Fresh parsley, chopped (optional for garnish)

Instructions:

1. Place the eggs in a single layer in a saucepan or pot.
2. Add enough water to the pot to cover the eggs by at least an inch.
3. Place the pot on the stove over medium heat and bring the water to a boil.
4. Once boiling, reduce the heat to a simmer and let the eggs cook for 9-12 minutes depending on your desired yolk consistency (9 minutes for soft-boiled, 12 minutes for hard-boiled).
5. While the eggs are cooking, prepare an ice bath by filling a bowl with cold water and ice cubes.
6. Once the eggs are cooked to your liking, carefully transfer them to the ice bath to cool rapidly. Let them sit for a few minutes.
7. Once the eggs are cooled, gently tap them on a hard surface to crack the shell, then peel the shell off.
8. Cut the hard-boiled eggs in half and sprinkle paprika, salt, and pepper over the yolks.
9. Optionally, garnish with chopped fresh parsley for added freshness.
10. Serve and enjoy your hard-boiled eggs with paprika as a snack or appetizer.

Appetizers

Caprese Skewers:

Ingredients:

- Cherry tomatoes
- Fresh mozzarella balls (bocconcini)
- Fresh basil leaves

- Extra-virgin olive oil
- Balsamic glaze
- Salt and pepper, to taste
- Wooden skewers

Instructions:

1. Rinse the cherry tomatoes and basil leaves. Drain any excess water.
2. Assemble the skewers by alternating cherry tomatoes, fresh mozzarella balls and fresh basil leaves onto the wooden skewers.
3. Arrange the assembled Caprese skewers on a serving platter.
4. Drizzle extra-virgin olive oil over the skewers.
5. Lightly sprinkle salt and pepper to taste.
6. Finish by drizzling balsamic glaze over the skewers for a burst of flavor.
7. Serve immediately and enjoy these delightful Caprese skewers as a refreshing appetizer or snack.

Stuffed Mushrooms with Spinach and Feta:

Ingredients:

- 24 large mushrooms, cleaned and stems removed
- 2 cups fresh spinach, chopped
- 1 cup feta cheese, crumbled
- 1/2 cup breadcrumbs
- 1/4 cup grated Parmesan cheese
- 2 cloves garlic, minced
- 2 tablespoons olive oil
- 1 teaspoon dried oregano
- Salt and pepper to taste

Instructions:

1. Preheat your oven to 375°F (190°C).
2. Chop the mushroom stems finely.

3. In a skillet, heat olive oil over medium heat. Add minced garlic and saute until fragrant.

4. Add chopped mushroom stems and spinach to the skillet. Cook until the spinach wilts and the mushroom stems are tender. Season with salt, pepper and dried oregano.

5. In a bowl, combine the cooked spinach and mushroom mixture with feta cheese and breadcrumbs. Mix well.

6. Spoon the filling into each mushroom cap, pressing down gently.

7. Place the stuffed mushrooms on a baking sheet lined with parchment paper.

8. Sprinkle grated Parmesan cheese over the stuffed mushrooms.

9. Bake in the preheated oven for 20-25 minutes or until the mushrooms are tender and the tops are golden brown.

10. Remove from the oven and let them cool for a few minutes before serving.

Cucumber Bites with Smoked Salmon:

Ingredients:

- 2 large cucumbers, peeled and sliced into rounds
- 4 ounces (about 113g) smoked salmon, thinly sliced
- 1/2 cup cream cheese, softened
- 2 tablespoons fresh dill, chopped
- 1 tablespoon capers, drained
- 1 tablespoon lemon juice
- Salt and pepper to taste

Instructions:

1. In a bowl, mix the softened cream cheese, chopped fresh dill and lemon juice until well combined. Season with salt and pepper to taste.

2. Pat the cucumber slices dry with a paper towel to remove excess moisture.

3. Take each cucumber round and spread a small amount of the cream cheese mixture on top.

4. Place a slice of smoked salmon on each cucumber round, slightly folding or arranging it to fit.

5. Garnish each cucumber bite with a few capers.

6. Arrange the cucumber bites on a serving platter.

7. Optional: sprinkle additional fresh dill on top for extra flavor.

8. Chill in the refrigerator for about 30 minutes before serving to allow the flavors to meld.

Guacamole with Veggie Sticks:

Ingredients:

- 2 large cucumbers, peeled and sliced into rounds
- 4 ounces (about 113g) smoked salmon, thinly sliced
- 1/2 cup cream cheese, softened
- 2 tablespoons fresh dill, chopped
- 1 tablespoon capers, drained
- 1 tablespoon lemon juice
- Salt and pepper to taste

Instructions:

1. In a bowl, mix the softened cream cheese, chopped fresh dill and lemon juice until well combined. Season with salt and pepper to taste.

2. Pat the cucumber slices dry with a paper towel to remove excess moisture.

3. Take each cucumber round and spread a small amount of the cream cheese mixture on top.

4. Place a slice of smoked salmon on each cucumber round, slightly folding or arranging it to fit.

5. Garnish each cucumber bite with a few capers.

6. Arrange the cucumber bites on a serving platter.

7. Optional: sprinkle additional fresh dill on top for extra flavor.

8. Chill in the refrigerator for about 30 minutes before serving to allow the flavors to meld.

Tomato Bruschetta:

Ingredients:

- 4 to 5 ripe tomatoes, diced
- 1/4 cup fresh basil, chopped
- 3 cloves garlic, minced
- 2 tablespoons extra-virgin olive oil
- 1 teaspoon balsamic vinegar
- Salt and pepper to taste
- Baguette or Italian bread, sliced

Instructions:

1. In a bowl, combine diced tomatoes, chopped fresh basil, minced garlic, olive oil and balsamic vinegar.
2. Mix the ingredients well and season with salt and pepper to taste. Allow the mixture to sit for at least 15-20 minutes to let the flavors meld.
3. Preheat your oven broiler or grill.
4. Slice the baguette or Italian bread into 1/2-inch thick slices.
5. Place the bread slices on a baking sheet and toast under the broiler or on the grill for 1-2 minutes on each side, until they are lightly golden.
6. Once toasted, rub each bread slice with a garlic clove for added flavor.
7. Spoon the tomato mixture generously onto each toasted bread slice.
8. Serve the tomato bruschetta immediately.

Shrimp Cocktail:

Ingredients:

For the Shrimp:

- 1 pound (about 450g) large shrimp, peeled and deveined

- 1 tablespoon olive oil
- 1 teaspoon Old Bay seasoning (optional)
- Salt and pepper to taste

For the Cocktail Sauce:

- 1/2 cup ketchup
- 2 tablespoons horseradish (adjust to taste)
- 1 tablespoon fresh lemon juice
- 1 teaspoon Worcestershire sauce
- Dash of hot sauce (optional)
- Salt and pepper to taste

For Garnish:

- Fresh lemon wedges
- Fresh parsley, chopped

Instructions:

1. Preheat the oven to 400°F (200°C).
2. In a bowl, toss the peeled and deveined shrimp with olive oil, Old Bay seasoning (if using), salt and pepper.
3. Spread the seasoned shrimp on a baking sheet in a single layer.
4. Bake in the preheated oven for 8-10 minutes or until the shrimp are opaque and cooked through. Be careful not to overcook.
5. While the shrimp are baking, prepare the cocktail sauce. In a bowl, mix together ketchup, horseradish, fresh lemon juice, Worcestershire sauce, hot sauce (if using), salt and pepper. Adjust the horseradish to your desired level of spiciness.
6. Once the shrimp are done, let them cool for a few minutes.
7. Arrange the cooked shrimp on a serving platter with a bowl of the cocktail sauce in the center.
8. Garnish with fresh lemon wedges and chopped parsley.
9. Serve the shrimp cocktail immediately.

Quinoa-Stuffed Bell Peppers:

Ingredients:

- 4 large bell peppers, halved and seeds removed
- 1 cup quinoa, rinsed and cooked according to package instructions
- 1 can (15 ounces) black beans, drained and rinsed
- 1 cup corn kernels (fresh, frozen or canned)
- 1 cup cherry tomatoes, diced
- 1/2 cup red onion, finely chopped
- 1/2 cup fresh cilantro, chopped
- 1 teaspoon ground cumin
- 1 teaspoon chili powder
- Salt and pepper to taste
- 1 cup shredded cheese (cheddar, Monterey Jack or a blend)

Instructions:

1. Preheat your oven to 375°F (190°C).
2. Cook quinoa according to package instructions.
3. In a large mixing bowl, combine the cooked quinoa, black beans, corn, cherry tomatoes, red onion, cilantro, ground cumin, chili powder, salt and pepper. Mix well.
4. Place the halved bell peppers in a baking dish.
5. Spoon the quinoa mixture into each bell pepper half, pressing down gently.
6. Sprinkle shredded cheese over the top of each stuffed pepper.
7. Cover the baking dish with aluminum foil.
8. Bake in the preheated oven for 25-30 minutes or until the peppers are tender.
9. Remove the foil and bake for an additional 5-10 minutes, allowing the cheese to melt and turn golden.
10. Remove from the oven and let them cool for a few minutes before serving.

Smoked Almond and Cranberry Cheese Ball:

Ingredients:

- 8 ounces (about 225g) cream cheese, softened
- 1 cup sharp cheddar cheese, shredded
- 1/2 cup smoked almonds, finely chopped
- 1/2 cup dried cranberries, finely chopped
- 2 green onions, finely chopped
- 1 teaspoon Worcestershire sauce
- 1/2 teaspoon garlic powder
- Salt and pepper to taste
- 1/2 cup smoked almonds, coarsely chopped (for coating)

Instructions:

1. In a large bowl, combine the softened cream cheese and shredded cheddar cheese. Mix until smooth and well combined.
2. Add finely chopped smoked almonds, dried cranberries, green onions, Worcestershire sauce, garlic powder, salt and pepper to the cheese mixture. Mix thoroughly.
3. Shape the mixture into a ball and wrap it in plastic wrap.
4. Refrigerate the cheese ball for at least 1-2 hours to allow it to firm up.
5. After chilling, unwrap the cheese ball and roll it in the coarsely chopped smoked almonds, covering the entire surface.
6. Place the cheese ball on a serving platter.
7. Optional: Garnish with additional chopped cranberries, green onions or smoked almonds for a decorative touch.
8. Serve the smoked almond and cranberry cheese ball with crackers or sliced baguette.

Zucchini Roll-Ups with Hummus:

Ingredients:

- 2 medium zucchinis, thinly sliced lengthwise
- 1 cup hummus (store-bought or homemade)
- 1 cup cherry tomatoes, diced
- 1/2 cup cucumber, diced
- 1/4 cup red onion, finely chopped
- 2 tablespoons fresh parsley, chopped
- 1 tablespoon lemon juice
- Salt and pepper to taste

Instructions:

1. Preheat your oven to 375°F (190°C).
2. Place the zucchini slices on a baking sheet lined with parchment paper.
3. Lightly brush each zucchini slice with olive oil and season with salt and pepper.
4. Bake in the preheated oven for 8-10 minutes or until the zucchini slices are slightly softened. Allow them to cool.
5. In a bowl, mix together diced cherry tomatoes, cucumber, red onion, fresh parsley, and lemon juice. Season with salt and pepper to taste.
6. Spread a thin layer of hummus onto each zucchini slice.
7. Spoon the vegetable mixture over the hummus on each zucchini slice.
8. Carefully roll up each zucchini slice to create the roll-ups.
9. Secure with toothpicks if needed and place them on a serving platter.
10. Optional: Garnish with additional chopped parsley or a drizzle of olive oil.

Artichoke and Spinach Dip:

Ingredients:

- 1 (10-ounce) package frozen chopped spinach, thawed and drained
- 1 (14-ounce) can artichoke hearts, drained and chopped
- 1 cup mayonnaise
- 1 cup sour cream
- 1 cup grated Parmesan cheese

- 1 cup shredded mozzarella cheese

- 2 cloves garlic, minced

- 1 teaspoon dried oregano

- 1/2 teaspoon garlic powder

- Salt and pepper to taste

- Baguette slices, tortilla chips or vegetable sticks for serving

Instructions:

1. Preheat your oven to 375°F (190°C).

2. In a large mixing bowl, combine the thawed and drained chopped spinach with the chopped artichoke hearts.

3. Add mayonnaise, sour cream, grated Parmesan cheese, shredded mozzarella cheese, minced garlic, dried oregano, garlic powder, salt and pepper to the bowl. Mix until well combined.

4. Transfer the mixture to a baking dish, spreading it evenly.

5. Bake in the preheated oven for 25-30 minutes or until the dip is hot and bubbly and the top is golden brown.

6. Remove from the oven and let it cool for a few minutes before serving.

7. Serve the Artichoke and Spinach Dip with baguette slices, tortilla chips or vegetable sticks.

Deviled Eggs with Avocado:

Ingredients:

- 6 hard-boiled eggs, peeled and cut in half lengthwise

- 1 ripe avocado, peeled and pit removed

- 2 tablespoons mayonnaise

- 1 tablespoon Dijon mustard

- 1 tablespoon fresh lemon juice

- Salt and pepper to taste

- Paprika and fresh chives for garnish

Instructions:

1. Cut the hard-boiled eggs in half lengthwise and carefully remove the yolks. Place the yolks in a bowl.

2. In the same bowl, add the ripe avocado, mayonnaise, Dijon mustard and fresh lemon juice.

3. Mash and mix the ingredients together until smooth and well combined. You can also use a food processor for a smoother consistency.

4. Season the avocado and egg yolk mixture with salt and pepper to taste. Adjust the seasoning according to your preference.

5. Spoon or pipe the avocado and egg yolk mixture back into the egg white halves.

6. Sprinkle paprika over the filled deviled eggs for added flavor and a pop of color.

7. Garnish with fresh chives.

8. Refrigerate the deviled eggs for at least 30 minutes before serving to allow the flavors to meld.

Cauliflower Buffalo Bites:

Ingredients:

For the Cauliflower Bites:

- 1 medium cauliflower head, cut into florets
- 1 cup all-purpose flour
- 1 cup milk (dairy or plant-based)
- 1 teaspoon garlic powder
- 1 teaspoon onion powder
- 1/2 teaspoon smoked paprika
- Salt and pepper to taste

For the Buffalo Sauce:

- 1/2 cup hot sauce (like Frank's RedHot)
- 1/4 cup unsalted butter, melted
- 1 tablespoon honey (optional for sweetness)

- 1 teaspoon garlic powder
- 1 teaspoon Worcestershire sauce (optional)

Instructions:

1. Preheat your oven to 450°F (230°C). Line a baking sheet with parchment paper.
2. In a bowl, whisk together flour, milk, garlic powder, onion powder, smoked paprika, salt and pepper to create a batter.
3. Dip each cauliflower floret into the batter, ensuring it is well-coated and place it on the prepared baking sheet.
4. Bake the cauliflower in the preheated oven for 20-25 minutes or until golden brown and crispy, flipping halfway through.
5. While the cauliflower is baking, prepare the Buffalo sauce by whisking together hot sauce, melted butter, honey (if using) garlic powder and Worcestershire sauce in a bowl.
6. Once the cauliflower is done, transfer the florets to a large bowl and drizzle the Buffalo sauce over them. Toss until each floret is evenly coated.
7. Return the sauced cauliflower to the baking sheet and bake for an additional 10 minutes until the sauce is sticky and caramelized.
8. Remove from the oven and let them cool for a few minutes.

Herbed Greek Yogurt Dip:

Ingredients:

- 1 cup Greek yogurt
- 2 tablespoons fresh parsley, finely chopped
- 1 tablespoon fresh dill, finely chopped
- 1 tablespoon fresh mint, finely chopped
- 1 clove garlic, minced
- 1 tablespoon extra-virgin olive oil
- 1 teaspoon lemon juice
- Salt and pepper to taste

Instructions:

1. In a bowl, combine Greek yogurt, chopped parsley, chopped dill, chopped mint, minced garlic, olive oil and lemon juice.

2. Mix the ingredients together until well combined.

3. Season the herbed Greek yogurt dip with salt and pepper to taste. Adjust the seasoning according to your preference.

4. Cover the bowl with plastic wrap and refrigerate for at least 30 minutes to allow the flavors to meld.

5. Before serving, give the dip a quick stir.

6. Optional: Drizzle a bit of olive oil on top and garnish with additional chopped herbs for presentation.

7. Serve the herbed Greek yogurt dip with fresh vegetables, pita chips, or as a refreshing sauce for grilled meats.

Sweet Potato Rounds with Guacamole:

Ingredients:

For Sweet Potato Rounds:

- 2 large sweet potatoes, scrubbed and sliced into rounds
- 2 tablespoons olive oil
- 1 teaspoon smoked paprika
- 1/2 teaspoon garlic powder
- Salt and pepper to taste

For Guacamole:

- 2 ripe avocados, peeled and pitted
- 1 small tomato, diced
- 1/4 cup red onion, finely chopped
- 1 clove garlic, minced
- 1 tablespoon fresh cilantro, chopped
- 1 tablespoon lime juice

- Salt and pepper to taste

Instructions:

For Sweet Potato Rounds:

1. Preheat your oven to 400°F (200°C).
2. In a bowl, toss sweet potato rounds with olive oil, smoked paprika, garlic powder, salt and pepper until evenly coated.
3. Place the sweet potato rounds on a baking sheet in a single layer.
4. Bake in the preheated oven for 20-25 minutes, flipping halfway through or until the sweet potatoes are tender and lightly browned.

For Guacamole:

1. In a bowl, mash the ripe avocados with a fork.
2. Add diced tomato, chopped red onion, minced garlic, chopped cilantro, lime juice, salt and pepper to the mashed avocados. Mix until well combined.
3. Adjust the seasoning according to your taste preferences.

To Serve:

1. Arrange the baked sweet potato rounds on a serving platter.
2. Top each sweet potato round with a spoonful of guacamole.
3. Optional: Garnish with additional cilantro or a squeeze of lime juice.

Lemon Herb Marinated Olives:

Ingredients:

- 1 cup mixed olives (green and black), pitted
- 2 tablespoons extra-virgin olive oil
- Zest of 1 lemon
- 2 tablespoons fresh lemon juice
- 2 cloves garlic, minced
- 1 teaspoon fresh rosemary, finely chopped
- 1 teaspoon fresh thyme leaves
- 1/2 teaspoon dried oregano

- Pinch of red pepper flakes (optional)
- Salt and black pepper to taste

Instructions:

1. In a bowl, combine the mixed olives.
2. In a separate small bowl, whisk together the extra-virgin olive oil, lemon zest, lemon juice, minced garlic, chopped rosemary, thyme leaves, dried oregano, red pepper flakes (if using) salt and black pepper.
3. Pour the marinade over the olives, ensuring they are well coated. Toss gently to combine.
4. Cover the bowl with plastic wrap and let the olives marinate in the refrigerator for at least 1-2 hours or overnight for a more intense flavor.
5. Before serving, bring the olives to room temperature for about 30 minutes.
6. Optional: Garnish with additional fresh herbs or a drizzle of extra-virgin olive oil.

Kale and Quinoa Salad with Roasted Butternut Squash:

Ingredients:

For the Salad:

- 1 cup quinoa, rinsed and cooked according to package instructions
- 4 cups kale, stems removed and finely chopped
- 2 cups butternut squash, peeled and diced
- 1 tablespoon olive oil
- Salt and pepper to taste
- 1/2 cup dried cranberries
- 1/2 cup feta cheese, crumbled
- 1/4 cup pumpkin seeds (pepitas)

For the Dressing:

- 3 tablespoons extra-virgin olive oil
- 2 tablespoons apple cider vinegar
- 1 tablespoon Dijon mustard
- 1 tablespoon maple syrup
- Salt and pepper to taste

Instructions:

1. Preheat your oven to 400°F (200°C).
2. Toss the diced butternut squash in olive oil and season with salt and pepper. Spread it on a baking sheet in a single layer.
3. Roast the butternut squash in the preheated oven for 20-25 minutes or until tender and golden brown, stirring halfway through. Allow it to cool.
4. In a large bowl, combine cooked quinoa, finely chopped kale, roasted butternut squash, dried cranberries, crumbled feta cheese and pumpkin seeds.

5. In a small bowl, whisk together extra-virgin olive oil, apple cider vinegar, Dijon mustard, maple syrup, salt and pepper to create the dressing.

6. Pour the dressing over the salad and toss until all ingredients are well coated.

7. Let the salad sit for a few minutes to allow the flavors to meld.

8. Serve the Kale and Quinoa Salad with Roasted Butternut Squash at room temperature or chilled.

Citrus Avocado Salad with Shrimp:

Ingredients:

For the Shrimp:

- 1 pound large shrimp, peeled and deveined
- 2 tablespoons olive oil
- 1 teaspoon chili powder
- Salt and pepper to taste
- Zest of 1 lime

For the Salad:

- 4 cups mixed salad greens (spinach, arugula or your choice)
- 2 ripe avocados, peeled, pitted and sliced
- 1 grapefruit, segmented
- 2 oranges, segmented
- 1/4 cup red onion, thinly sliced
- 1/4 cup fresh cilantro, chopped

For the Citrus Vinaigrette:

- 1/4 cup extra-virgin olive oil
- 2 tablespoons fresh orange juice
- 1 tablespoon fresh lime juice
- 1 tablespoon honey
- Salt and pepper to taste

Instructions:

For the Shrimp:

1. In a bowl, combine shrimp with olive oil, chili powder, salt, pepper and lime zest.
2. Heat a skillet over medium-high heat. Add the shrimp and cook for 2-3 minutes per side or until they are pink and opaque. Set aside.

For the Salad:

1. In a large salad bowl, arrange the mixed greens.
2. Top the greens with sliced avocados, grapefruit segments, orange segments, sliced red onion and cooked shrimp.
3. Sprinkle chopped cilantro over the salad.

For the Citrus Vinaigrette:

1. In a small bowl, whisk together extra-virgin olive oil, fresh orange juice, fresh lime juice, honey, salt and pepper.
2. Drizzle the citrus vinaigrette over the salad just before serving.
3. Toss the salad gently to coat all ingredients with the dressing.

Asian-Inspired Cabbage Salad:

Ingredients:

For the Salad:

- 4 cups shredded cabbage (green or Napa)
- 1 cup shredded carrots
- 1 red bell pepper, thinly sliced
- 1/2 cup edamame, cooked and shelled
- 1/4 cup green onions, sliced
- 1/4 cup cilantro, chopped
- 1/4 cup peanuts or cashews, chopped (optional)

For the Dressing:

- 3 tablespoons soy sauce
- 2 tablespoons rice vinegar
- 1 tablespoon sesame oil

- 1 tablespoon honey or maple syrup
- 1 teaspoon fresh ginger, grated
- 1 clove garlic, minced
- 1 teaspoon sriracha or chili garlic sauce (optional)
- Sesame seeds for garnish

Instructions:

1. In a large bowl, combine shredded cabbage, shredded carrots, sliced red bell pepper, edamame, sliced green onions and chopped cilantro.
2. In a separate small bowl, whisk together soy sauce, rice vinegar, sesame oil, honey or maple syrup, grated ginger, minced garlic and sriracha (if using).
3. Pour the dressing over the salad and toss to coat the vegetables evenly.
4. Let the salad marinate in the refrigerator for at least 15-20 minutes to enhance the flavors.
5. Before serving, sprinkle chopped peanuts or cashews (if using) and sesame seeds over the salad.
6. Toss the salad once more and adjust the seasoning if needed.
7. Serve the Asian-Inspired Cabbage Salad as a side dish or add protein like grilled chicken or tofu for a complete meal.

Watermelon Feta Salad with Mint:

Ingredients:

- 4 cups seedless watermelon, cubed
- 1 cup feta cheese, crumbled
- 1/4 cup fresh mint leaves, chopped
- 2 tablespoons extra-virgin olive oil
- 1 tablespoon balsamic vinegar
- Salt and black pepper to taste

Instructions:

1. In a large serving bowl, combine the cubed watermelon, crumbled feta cheese and chopped fresh mint.
2. Drizzle extra-virgin olive oil and balsamic vinegar over the watermelon, feta and mint.
3. Gently toss the ingredients to coat them evenly with the dressing.
4. Season the salad with salt and black pepper to taste. Be mindful of the saltiness of the feta when adding salt.
5. Optional: Garnish with additional mint leaves for a fresh and vibrant presentation.
6. Refrigerate the Watermelon Feta Salad for about 15-30 minutes before serving to allow the flavors to meld.

Mango Black Bean Salad:

Ingredients:

- 2 ripe mangoes, peeled, pitted and diced
- 1 can (15 ounces) black beans, drained and rinsed
- 1 cup cherry tomatoes, halved
- 1/2 cup red bell pepper, diced
- 1/4 cup red onion, finely chopped
- 1/4 cup fresh cilantro, chopped
- 1 jalapeño, seeds removed and finely chopped (optional, for heat)

For the Dressing:

- 2 tablespoons lime juice
- 2 tablespoons extra-virgin olive oil
- 1 teaspoon honey or maple syrup
- 1/2 teaspoon ground cumin
- Salt and black pepper to taste

Instructions:

1. In a large bowl, combine diced mangoes, black beans, halved cherry tomatoes, diced red bell pepper, chopped red onion, cilantro and chopped jalapeño (if using).

2. In a small bowl, whisk together lime juice, extra-virgin olive oil, honey or maple syrup, ground cumin, salt and black pepper to create the dressing.

3. Pour the dressing over the mango and black bean mixture.

4. Gently toss the salad until all ingredients are well coated with the dressing.

5. Let the Mango Black Bean Salad sit for a few minutes to allow the flavors to meld.

6. Optional: Garnish with additional cilantro before serving.

7. Serve the salad as a side dish, on top of grilled chicken or fish or with tortilla chips.

Arugula Pomegranate Salad with Goat Cheese:

Ingredients:

- 4 cups arugula, washed and dried
- 1 cup pomegranate arils (seeds)
- 1/2 cup crumbled goat cheese
- 1/4 cup chopped walnuts or pecans, toasted
- 2 tablespoons extra-virgin olive oil
- 1 tablespoon balsamic vinegar
- 1 teaspoon honey
- Salt and black pepper to taste

Instructions:

1. In a large salad bowl, combine arugula, pomegranate arils, crumbled goat cheese and toasted nuts.

2. In a small bowl, whisk together extra-virgin olive oil, balsamic vinegar, honey, salt, and black pepper to create the dressing.

3. Pour the dressing over the arugula, pomegranate and goat cheese mixture.

4. Gently toss the salad until the ingredients are evenly coated with the dressing.

5. Let the Arugula Pomegranate Salad sit for a few minutes to allow the flavors to mingle.

6. Serve the salad as a refreshing side dish or add grilled chicken or salmon for a complete meal.

Spinach Strawberry Salad with Balsamic Reduction:

Ingredients:

For the Salad:

- 6 cups baby spinach, washed and dried
- 1 1/2 cups fresh strawberries, hulled and sliced
- 1/2 cup sliced almonds, toasted
- 1/4 cup red onion, thinly sliced
- 1/4 cup feta cheese, crumbled

For the Balsamic Reduction:

- 1/2 cup balsamic vinegar
- 2 tablespoons honey or maple syrup

For the Dressing:

- 3 tablespoons extra-virgin olive oil
- Salt and black pepper to taste

Instructions:

For the Balsamic Reduction:

1. In a small saucepan, combine balsamic vinegar and honey (or maple syrup).
2. Bring the mixture to a simmer over medium heat.
3. Reduce the heat to low and let it simmer for 10-15 minutes or until the vinegar has thickened and reduced by about half. Stir occasionally.
4. Remove from heat and let it cool. The reduction will continue to thicken as it cools.

For the Salad:

1. In a large salad bowl, combine baby spinach, sliced strawberries, toasted sliced almonds, sliced red onion and crumbled feta cheese.

2. In a small bowl, whisk together extra-virgin olive oil, salt and black pepper to create the dressing.

3. Drizzle the dressing over the salad and toss gently to coat the ingredients evenly.

4. Drizzle the balsamic reduction over the salad just before serving. Use as much or as little as you prefer.

5. Toss the salad once more to incorporate the balsamic reduction.

6. Serve the Spinach Strawberry Salad with Balsamic Reduction as a delightful and flavorful side dish.

Roasted Brussels Sprouts and Sweet Potato Salad:

Ingredients:

For the Salad:

- 1 pound Brussels sprouts, trimmed and halved
- 2 medium sweet potatoes, peeled and diced
- 2 tablespoons olive oil
- Salt and black pepper to taste
- 1/2 cup pecans, chopped and toasted
- 1/4 cup dried cranberries
- 1/4 cup feta cheese, crumbled
- 2 tablespoons fresh parsley, chopped

For the Dressing:

- 3 tablespoons balsamic vinegar
- 2 tablespoons extra-virgin olive oil
- 1 tablespoon Dijon mustard
- 1 tablespoon maple syrup
- Salt and black pepper to taste

Instructions:

1. Preheat your oven to 400°F (200°C).

2. In a large mixing bowl, toss Brussels sprouts and diced sweet potatoes with olive oil, salt and black pepper until well coated.

3. Spread the vegetables in a single layer on a baking sheet.

4. Roast in the preheated oven for 20-25 minutes or until the Brussels sprouts are golden brown and the sweet potatoes are tender stirring halfway through.

5. While the vegetables are roasting, prepare the dressing. In a small bowl, whisk together balsamic vinegar, extra-virgin olive oil, Dijon mustard, maple syrup, salt and black pepper.

6. Once the vegetables are done transfer them to a large salad bowl.

7. Add chopped and toasted pecans, dried cranberries, crumbled feta cheese and fresh parsley to the bowl.

8. Drizzle the dressing over the salad and toss gently to combine all the ingredients.

9. Adjust salt and pepper to taste.

10. Serve the Roasted Brussels Sprouts and Sweet Potato Salad warm or at room temperature.

Caprese Salad with Avocado:

Ingredients:

- 4 large tomatoes, sliced
- 2 ripe avocados, sliced
- 1/2 pound fresh mozzarella cheese, sliced
- Fresh basil leaves
- Extra-virgin olive oil
- Balsamic glaze
- Salt and black pepper to taste

Instructions:

1. Arrange the tomato slices, avocado slices, and fresh mozzarella cheese on a serving platter, alternating them for a visually appealing presentation.

2. Tuck fresh basil leaves in between the slices.

3. Drizzle extra-virgin olive oil over the tomato, avocado and mozzarella slices.

4. Lightly season the salad with salt and black pepper to taste.

5. Finish the Caprese Salad with Avocado by drizzling balsamic glaze over the top.

6. Serve immediately and enjoy the vibrant flavors of this classic salad with a creamy twist.

Mediterranean Orzo Salad:

Ingredients:

For the Salad:

- 1 cup orzo pasta, cooked according to package instructions and cooled
- 1 cup cherry tomatoes, halved
- 1 cucumber, diced
- 1/2 red bell pepper, diced
- 1/4 red onion, finely chopped
- 1/2 cup Kalamata olives, sliced
- 1/2 cup feta cheese, crumbled
- 1/4 cup fresh parsley, chopped

For the Dressing:

- 3 tablespoons extra-virgin olive oil
- 2 tablespoons red wine vinegar
- 1 teaspoon Dijon mustard
- 1 clove garlic, minced
- 1 teaspoon dried oregano
- Salt and black pepper to taste

Instructions:

1. Cook the orzo pasta according to package instructions. Once cooked, drain and let it cool.

2. In a large bowl, combine the cooked and cooled orzo pasta with halved cherry tomatoes, diced cucumber, diced red bell pepper, finely chopped red onion, sliced Kalamata olives, crumbled feta cheese and chopped fresh parsley.

3. In a small bowl, whisk together extra-virgin olive oil, red wine vinegar, Dijon mustard, minced garlic, dried oregano, salt and black pepper to create the dressing.

4. Pour the dressing over the orzo salad and toss gently until all ingredients are well coated.

5. Refrigerate the Mediterranean Orzo Salad for at least 30 minutes before serving to let the flavors meld.

6. Before serving, toss the salad once more and adjust the seasoning if needed.

7. Serve the orzo salad as a refreshing and satisfying side dish or light meal.

Thai-Inspired Zucchini Noodle Salad:

Ingredients:

For the Zucchini Noodles:

- 4 medium zucchinis, spiralized into noodles
- Salt for sprinkling

For the Salad:

- 1 cup shredded carrots
- 1 red bell pepper, thinly sliced
- 1 cup bean sprouts
- 1/4 cup chopped fresh cilantro
- 1/4 cup chopped fresh mint
- 1/4 cup chopped peanuts
- Lime wedges for serving

For the Dressing:

- 3 tablespoons soy sauce
- 2 tablespoons lime juice
- 1 tablespoon sesame oil

- 1 tablespoon honey or agave nectar
- 1 teaspoon fresh ginger, grated
- 1 clove garlic, minced
- 1 teaspoon Sriracha or chili garlic sauce (adjust to taste)

Instructions:

1. Spiralize a zucchini into noodles. Sprinkle the zucchini noodles with salt and let them sit for about 15-20 minutes to release excess moisture. Afterward pat them dry with a paper towel.

2. In a large bowl, combine the zucchini noodles with shredded carrots, thinly sliced red bell pepper, bean sprouts, chopped cilantro, chopped mint and chopped peanuts.

3. In a small bowl, whisk together soy sauce, lime juice, sesame oil, honey or agave nectar, grated ginger, minced garlic and Sriracha.

4. Pour the dressing over the zucchini noodle salad and toss gently to coat the ingredients evenly.

5. Let the Thai-inspired Zucchini Noodle Salad sit for a few minutes to allow the flavors to meld.

6. Serve the salad with lime wedges on the side for an extra burst of freshness.

Cucumber and Radish Salad with Dill Yogurt Dressing:

Ingredients:

For the Salad:

- 2 large cucumbers, thinly sliced
- 1 bunch radishes, thinly sliced
- 1/4 cup red onion, thinly sliced
- 2 tablespoons fresh dill, chopped
- Salt and black pepper to taste

For the Dill Yogurt Dressing:

- 1 cup Greek yogurt

- 2 tablespoons fresh dill, chopped
- 1 tablespoon lemon juice
- 1 tablespoon extra-virgin olive oil
- 1 clove garlic, minced
- Salt and black pepper to taste

Instructions:

1. In a large bowl, combine the thinly sliced cucumbers, radishes, red onion and chopped fresh dill.
2. Sprinkle salt and black pepper over the vegetables and toss gently to combine. Let it sit for a few minutes to allow the salt to draw out some moisture from the cucumbers.
3. In a separate bowl, whisk together Greek yogurt, chopped dill, lemon juice, extra-virgin olive oil, minced garlic, salt and black pepper to create the dressing.
4. Pour the dill yogurt dressing over the cucumber and radish mixture.
5. Toss the salad gently until the vegetables are evenly coated with the dressing.
6. Refrigerate the Cucumber and Radish Salad for about 15-30 minutes before serving to allow the flavors to meld.
7. Before serving, give the salad a quick stir.
8. Optional: Garnish with additional chopped dill for a fresh touch.

Quinoa and Mango Tango Salad:

Ingredients:

For the Salad:

- 1 cup quinoa, rinsed and cooked according to package instructions
- 1 large mango, peeled, pitted, and diced
- 1 cup cucumber, diced
- 1/2 cup red bell pepper, diced
- 1/4 cup red onion, finely chopped
- 1/4 cup fresh cilantro, chopped

- 1/4 cup toasted almonds, chopped

For the Dressing:

- 3 tablespoons extra-virgin olive oil
- 2 tablespoons lime juice
- 1 tablespoon honey or agave nectar
- 1 teaspoon ground cumin
- Salt and black pepper to taste

Instructions:

1. Cook the quinoa according to package instructions and let it cool to room temperature.
2. In a large bowl, combine the cooked quinoa with diced mango, diced cucumber, diced red bell pepper, chopped red onion, chopped cilantro and chopped toasted almonds.
3. In a small bowl, whisk together extra-virgin olive oil, lime juice, honey or agave nectar, ground cumin, salt and black pepper to create the dressing.
4. Pour the dressing over the quinoa and mango mixture.
5. Toss the salad gently until all ingredients are well coated with the dressing.
6. Refrigerate the Quinoa and Mango Tango Salad for at least 30 minutes before serving to let the flavors meld.
7. Before serving, give the salad a quick stir.
8. Serve as a side dish or enjoy it on its own for a light and nutritious meal.

Beet and Goat Cheese Salad with Walnuts:

Ingredients:

For the Salad:

- 4 medium beets, roasted, peeled, and sliced
- 4 cups mixed salad greens (arugula, spinach or your choice)
- 1/2 cup goat cheese, crumbled
- 1/2 cup walnuts, toasted and chopped

For the Dressing:

- 3 tablespoons balsamic vinegar
- 2 tablespoons extra-virgin olive oil
- 1 tablespoon honey
- Salt and black pepper to taste

Instructions:

1. Preheat your oven to 400°F (200°C).
2. Wrap the beets individually in aluminum foil and roast them in the preheated oven for about 45-60 minutes or until they are tender when pierced with a fork. Let them cool, then peel and slice into rounds.
3. In a large salad bowl, combine the sliced roasted beets with mixed salad greens.
4. Sprinkle crumbled goat cheese and chopped toasted walnuts over the salad.
5. In a small bowl, whisk together balsamic vinegar, extra-virgin olive oil, honey, salt and black pepper to create the dressing.
6. Drizzle the dressing over the beet, goat cheese and walnut salad.
7. Toss the salad gently until all ingredients are well coated with the dressing.
8. Refrigerate the Beet and Goat Cheese Salad for about 15-30 minutes before serving to allow the flavors to meld.
9. Before serving, give the salad a quick stir.
10. Optional: Garnish with additional crumbled goat cheese and a sprinkle of toasted walnuts.

Protein-Packed Lentil Salad:

Ingredients:

For the Salad:

- 1 cup dry green or brown lentils, rinsed
- 3 cups water
- 1 cucumber, diced
- 1 red bell pepper, diced

- 1/2 red onion, finely chopped
- 1 cup cherry tomatoes, halved
- 1/4 cup fresh parsley, chopped
- 1/4 cup feta cheese, crumbled (optional)
- Salt and black pepper to taste

For the Dressing:

- 3 tablespoons extra-virgin olive oil
- 2 tablespoons red wine vinegar
- 1 teaspoon Dijon mustard
- 1 clove garlic, minced
- 1/2 teaspoon dried oregano
- Salt and black pepper to taste

Instructions:

1. In a medium saucepan, combine rinsed lentils and water. Bring to a boil, then reduce the heat to low and simmer for about 20-25 minutes or until lentils are tender but still have a slight bite. Drain any excess water.
2. In a large bowl, combine cooked lentils, diced cucumber, diced red bell pepper, finely chopped red onion, cherry tomatoes, chopped fresh parsley and crumbled feta cheese (if using).
3. In a small bowl, whisk together extra-virgin olive oil, red wine vinegar, Dijon mustard, minced garlic, dried oregano, salt and black pepper to create the dressing.
4. Pour the dressing over the lentil salad and toss gently to coat the ingredients evenly.
5. Season the salad with additional salt and black pepper to taste.
6. Refrigerate the Protein-Packed Lentil Salad for about 30 minutes before serving to let the flavors meld.
7. Before serving, give the salad a quick stir.
8. Serve the salad as a satisfying and protein-rich meal or as a side dish.

Desserts with a Twist

Avocado Chocolate Mousse:

Ingredients:

- 2 ripe avocados, peeled and pitted
- 1/2 cup unsweetened cocoa powder
- 1/2 cup maple syrup or agave nectar
- 1/4 cup almond milk or any milk of your choice
- 1 teaspoon vanilla extract
- Pinch of salt
- Optional toppings: whipped cream, berries, chopped nuts

Instructions:

1. In a food processor or blender, combine the ripe avocados, cocoa powder, maple syrup or agave nectar, almond milk, vanilla extract and a pinch of salt.
2. Blend the ingredients until smooth and creamy, scraping down the sides as needed to ensure everything is well incorporated.
3. Taste the chocolate mousse and adjust sweetness if necessary by adding more maple syrup or agave nectar.
4. Once the mixture is smooth and sweetened to your liking, transfer the chocolate mousse to serving bowls or glasses.
5. Refrigerate the Avocado Chocolate Mousse for at least 1-2 hours to allow it to chill and set.
6. Before serving, you can top the mousse with whipped cream, fresh berries, or chopped nuts for added texture and flavor.
7. Enjoy this creamy and indulgent Avocado Chocolate Mousse as a healthier alternative to traditional chocolate mousse!

Chia Seed Berry Parfait:

Ingredients:

For the Chia Seed Pudding:

- 1/4 cup chia seeds
- 1 cup almond milk or any milk of your choice
- 1 tablespoon maple syrup or honey
- 1/2 teaspoon vanilla extract

For the Berry Compote:

- 1 cup mixed berries (strawberries, blueberries, raspberries)
- 1 tablespoon maple syrup or honey
- 1 tablespoon water
- 1/2 teaspoon lemon zest (optional)

For the Parfait:

- Chia seed pudding
- Berry compote
- Greek yogurt or dairy-free yogurt
- Granola (optional)

Instructions:

For the Chia Seed Pudding:

1. In a bowl, combine chia seeds, almond milk, maple syrup or honey, and vanilla extract.
2. Whisk the ingredients together, ensuring that the chia seeds are evenly distributed.
3. Let the mixture sit for 5 minutes, then whisk again to prevent clumping.
4. Cover the bowl and refrigerate the chia seed pudding for at least 2 hours or overnight, allowing it to thicken.

For the Berry Compote:

1. In a small saucepan, combine mixed berries, maple syrup or honey, water and lemon zest (if using).
2. Bring the mixture to a gentle simmer over medium heat.
3. Cook the berries for 5-7 minutes or until they break down and release their juices, stirring occasionally.

4. Once the compote has thickened slightly, remove it from the heat and let it cool.

For the Parfait Assembly:

1. In serving glasses or jars, layer the chia seed pudding, berry compote and Greek yogurt.

2. Repeat the layers until the glass is filled, finishing with a dollop of Greek yogurt on top.

3. Optional: Sprinkle granola over the yogurt layer for added crunch.

4. Repeat the assembly for additional servings.

5. Chill the Chia Seed Berry Parfait in the refrigerator for at least 30 minutes before serving.

6. Garnish with fresh berries or mint leaves if desired.

Lemon Blueberry Quinoa Bars:

Ingredients:

For the Quinoa Crust:

- 1 cup cooked quinoa, cooled
- 1/4 cup almond flour
- 2 tablespoons coconut oil, melted
- 2 tablespoons maple syrup
- 1/2 teaspoon vanilla extract
- Pinch of salt

For the Lemon Blueberry Filling:

- 1 cup blueberries (fresh or frozen)
- 2 tablespoons lemon juice
- 1 teaspoon lemon zest
- 2 tablespoons maple syrup
- 1 tablespoon chia seeds

For the Crumb Topping:

- 2 tablespoons rolled oats

- 1 tablespoon almond flour
- 1 tablespoon coconut oil, melted
- 1 tablespoon maple syrup

Instructions:

For the Quinoa Crust:

1. Preheat the oven to 350°F (175°C) and line a baking dish with parchment paper.
2. In a bowl, combine cooked quinoa, almond flour, melted coconut oil, maple syrup, vanilla extract and a pinch of salt.
3. Press the mixture into the bottom of the prepared baking dish to form an even crust.
4. Bake the quinoa crust in the preheated oven for 15-18 minutes or until it becomes golden brown. Allow it to cool while preparing the filling.

For the Lemon Blueberry Filling:

1. In a small saucepan, combine blueberries, lemon juice, lemon zest and maple syrup.
2. Bring the mixture to a simmer over medium heat, stirring occasionally.
3. Once the blueberries break down and release their juices, stir in chia seeds and cook for an additional 2-3 minutes until the mixture thickens.
4. Remove the saucepan from the heat and let the lemon blueberry filling cool slightly.

For the Crumb Topping:

1. In a small bowl, combine rolled oats, almond flour, melted coconut oil and maple syrup to create the crumb topping.

Assembly:

1. Spread the lemon blueberry filling evenly over the cooled quinoa crust.
2. Sprinkle the crumb topping over the lemon blueberry layer.
3. Bake the bars in the oven for an additional 15-18 minutes or until the crumb topping is golden brown.

4. Allow the Lemon Blueberry Quinoa Bars to cool completely before slicing into squares or bars.

5. Optional: Garnish with additional lemon zest or a drizzle of maple syrup.

Coconut Mango Sorbet:

Ingredients:

- 2 cups ripe mango, peeled and diced
- 1 can (14 ounces) coconut milk
- 1/2 cup granulated sugar
- 1 tablespoon lime juice
- Pinch of salt
- Shredded coconut for garnish (optional)

Instructions:

1. Place the diced mango in a blender or food processor and blend until smooth.

2. In a saucepan over medium heat, combine coconut milk, granulated sugar, lime juice and a pinch of salt. Stir until the sugar is completely dissolved.

3. Remove the saucepan from heat and let the coconut milk mixture cool to room temperature.

4. Once cooled, combine the coconut milk mixture with the pureed mango in the blender or food processor. Blend until well combined.

5. Pour the mixture into a bowl and cover. Refrigerate for at least 3-4 hours or until thoroughly chilled.

6. Once chilled, transfer the mixture to an ice cream maker and churn according to the manufacturer's instructions.

7. Transfer the sorbet to a lidded container and freeze for an additional 3-4 hours or until firm.

8. Before serving, let the Coconut Mango Sorbet sit at room temperature for a few minutes to soften slightly.

9. Optional: Garnish with shredded coconut before serving.

10. Scoop and enjoy this refreshing Coconut Mango Sorbet as a tropical treat!

Greek Yogurt Berry Popsicles:

Ingredients:

- 1 cup Greek yogurt
- 1 cup mixed berries (strawberries, blueberries, raspberries)
- 2 tablespoons honey or maple syrup
- 1 teaspoon vanilla extract

Instructions:

1. In a blender or food processor, combine Greek yogurt, mixed berries, honey or maple syrup and vanilla extract.
2. Blend the ingredients until smooth and well combined.
3. Optional: If you prefer a chunkier texture, you can pulse the mixture briefly to leave some berry pieces.
4. Taste the mixture and adjust sweetness if needed by adding more honey or maple syrup.
5. Pour the yogurt and berry mixture into popsicle molds.
6. Insert popsicle sticks into each mold, making sure they are centered.
7. Freeze the Greek Yogurt Berry Popsicles for at least 4-6 hours or until fully set.
8. Once the popsicles are frozen, run the molds briefly under warm water to help release the popsicles.
9. Remove the popsicles from the molds and enjoy these refreshing and nutritious treats!

Pistachio and Matcha Energy Bites:

Ingredients:

- 1 cup rolled oats
- 1/2 cup shelled pistachios
- 2 tablespoons matcha powder

- 1/2 cup Medjool dates, pitted
- 1/4 cup honey or maple syrup
- 1 teaspoon vanilla extract
- Pinch of salt
- Shredded coconut for rolling (optional)

Instructions:

1. In a food processor, combine rolled oats, shelled pistachios and matcha powder. Pulse until the mixture resembles a coarse flour.
2. Add pitted Medjool dates, honey or maple syrup, vanilla extract and a pinch of salt to the food processor. Process until the mixture comes together and forms a sticky dough.
3. Taste the mixture and adjust sweetness if needed by adding more honey or maple syrup.
4. Scoop out tablespoon-sized portions of the mixture and roll them into balls using your hands.
5. Optional: Roll the energy bites in shredded coconut for added texture.
6. Place the Pistachio and Matcha Energy Bites on a parchment-lined tray and refrigerate for at least 30 minutes to firm up.
7. Once firm, transfer the energy bites to an airtight container and store them in the refrigerator for up to one week.
8. Enjoy these nutritious and flavorful Pistachio and Matcha Energy Bites as a quick and energizing snack!

Grilled Pineapple with Honey and Mint:

Ingredients:

- 1 pineapple, peeled, cored and cut into rings or spears
- 2 tablespoons honey
- Fresh mint leaves, chopped (for garnish)
- Optional: Vanilla ice cream or yogurt for serving

1. Preheat your grill to medium-high heat.

2. Place the pineapple rings or spears on the hot grill grates.

3. Grill the pineapple for 2-3 minutes per side or until it develops grill marks and caramelizes slightly.

4. During the last minute of grilling, brush each side of the pineapple with honey, allowing it to glaze and enhance the sweetness.

5. Remove the grilled pineapple from the grill and transfer it to a serving platter.

6. Drizzle any remaining honey over the grilled pineapple.

7. Garnish with chopped fresh mint leaves for a burst of freshness.

8. Optional: Serve the Grilled Pineapple with a scoop of vanilla ice cream or a dollop of yogurt for a delightful dessert.

9. Enjoy the sweet and smoky flavors of this Grilled Pineapple with Honey and Mint!

Chocolate-Dipped Strawberries with Almond Butter:

Ingredients:

- Fresh strawberries, washed and dried
- Dark chocolate, chopped (about 1 cup)
- 2 tablespoons almond butter
- Chopped almonds (optional for garnish)

Instructions:

1. In a heatproof bowl, melt the dark chocolate using a double boiler or microwave in 20-second intervals, stirring until smooth.

2. Stir almond butter into the melted chocolate until well combined.

3. Hold each strawberry by the stem and dip it into the chocolate-almond butter mixture, ensuring it's coated evenly.

4. Allow any excess chocolate to drip off, then place the chocolate-dipped strawberry on a parchment-lined tray.

5. Optional: Sprinkle chopped almonds over the chocolate while it's still wet for added crunch and flavor.

6. Repeat the process with the remaining strawberries.

7. Place the tray of Chocolate-Dipped Strawberries with Almond Butter in the refrigerator for about 30 minutes or until the chocolate sets.

8. Once the chocolate is firm, transfer the strawberries to a serving plate.

9. Serve as a delightful dessert or sweet treat.

Rosewater Watermelon Salad:

Ingredients:

- 4 cups watermelon, diced into bite-sized pieces
- 1 cucumber, peeled and diced
- 1/4 cup fresh mint leaves, chopped
- 1 tablespoon rosewater
- 1 tablespoon honey
- Juice of 1 lime
- 1/4 cup crumbled feta cheese (optional)
- Edible rose petals for garnish (optional)

Instructions:

1. In a large bowl, combine diced watermelon and peeled, diced cucumber.

2. In a small bowl, whisk together rosewater, honey and lime juice to create the dressing.

3. Pour the rosewater dressing over the watermelon and cucumber mixture. Toss gently to coat the fruit evenly.

4. Sprinkle chopped mint leaves over the salad and toss again to distribute the mint throughout.

5. Optional: Add crumbled feta cheese to the salad for a savory element. Toss lightly.

6. Refrigerate the Rosewater Watermelon Salad for about 15-30 minutes before serving to allow the flavors to meld.

7. Before serving, give the salad a quick stir.

8. Optional: Garnish with edible rose petals for a touch of elegance.

9. Serve this refreshing and fragrant Rosewater Watermelon Salad as a light side dish or a unique dessert.

Baked Apples with Cinnamon and Pecans:

Ingredients:

- 4 large apples (such as Honeycrisp or Granny Smith)
- 1/4 cup chopped pecans
- 2 tablespoons brown sugar
- 1 teaspoon ground cinnamon
- 2 tablespoons unsalted butter, melted
- 1/2 cup apple cider or water
- Vanilla ice cream or whipped cream for serving (optional)

Instructions:

1. Preheat your oven to 375°F (190°C).

2. Wash and core the apples, leaving the bottoms intact to form a well for the filling.

3. In a bowl, combine chopped pecans, brown sugar, ground cinnamon and melted butter. Mix until the ingredients are well incorporated.

4. Stuff each cored apple with the pecan mixture, pressing it down gently.

5. Place the stuffed apples in a baking dish.

6. Pour apple cider or water into the bottom of the baking dish to prevent the apples from sticking and to add moisture during baking.

7. Bake the apples in the preheated oven for 25-30 minutes or until they are tender but not mushy.

8. Optional: Baste the apples with some of the liquid in the baking dish halfway through the baking time.

9. Remove the baked apples from the oven and let them cool slightly.

10. Serve the Baked Apples with Cinnamon and Pecans warm, optionally topped with a scoop of vanilla ice cream or a dollop of whipped cream.

Tahini Date Truffles:

Ingredients:

- 1 cup dates, pitted
- 1/2 cup tahini
- 1/2 cup shredded coconut (plus extra for rolling)
- 1/4 cup almond flour
- 1/2 teaspoon vanilla extract
- Pinch of salt
- Optional: Crushed nuts or sesame seeds for coating

Instructions:

1. In a food processor, combine pitted dates, tahini, shredded coconut, almond flour, vanilla extract and a pinch of salt.
2. Process the mixture until it forms a sticky dough-like consistency.
3. If the mixture is too sticky, you can add more almond flour in small increments until it's easier to handle.
4. Scoop out tablespoon-sized portions of the mixture and roll them into balls using your hands.
5. Optional: Roll the tahini date truffles in shredded coconut, crushed nuts or sesame seeds for coating.
6. Place the truffles on a parchment-lined tray.
7. Refrigerate the Tahini Date Truffles for at least 30 minutes to firm up.
8. Once firm, transfer the truffles to an airtight container and store them in the refrigerator.
9. Serve and enjoy these delicious and nutritious Tahini Date Truffles as a sweet snack or dessert.

Orange and Almond Cake:

Ingredients:

For the Cake:

- 1 cup almond flour
- 1 cup all-purpose flour
- 1 cup granulated sugar
- 1 teaspoon baking powder
- 1/2 teaspoon baking soda
- 1/4 teaspoon salt
- 3 large eggs
- 1/2 cup unsalted butter, melted
- 1/2 cup plain Greek yogurt
- 1/3 cup fresh orange juice
- Zest of 2 oranges
- 1 teaspoon vanilla extract

For the Orange Glaze:

- 1 cup powdered sugar
- 2-3 tablespoons fresh orange juice
- Sliced almonds for garnish (optional)

Instructions:

1. Preheat your oven to 350°F (175°C). Grease and flour a round cake pan.
2. In a large bowl, whisk together almond flour, all-purpose flour, granulated sugar, baking powder, baking soda and salt.
3. In a separate bowl, beat the eggs. Add melted butter, Greek yogurt, fresh orange juice, orange zest and vanilla extract. Mix until well combined.
4. Pour the wet ingredients into the dry ingredients and stir until just combined. Do not overmix.
5. Pour the batter into the prepared cake pan and spread it evenly.

6. Bake in the preheated oven for 30-35 minutes or until a toothpick inserted into the center comes out clean.

7. While the cake is baking, prepare the orange glaze. In a bowl, whisk together powdered sugar and enough fresh orange juice to create a smooth glaze.

8. Once the cake is done, let it cool in the pan for 10 minutes then transfer it to a wire rack to cool completely.

9. Drizzle the orange glaze over the cooled cake.

10. Optional: Garnish with sliced almonds for added texture.

11. Slice and serve this moist and flavorful Orange and Almond Cake.

Matcha Green Tea Cheesecake Bites:

Ingredients:

For the Crust:

- 1 cup almond flour
- 2 tablespoons coconut oil, melted
- 1 tablespoon maple syrup
- Pinch of salt

For the Matcha Cheesecake Filling:

- 2 cups cream cheese, softened
- 1/2 cup powdered sugar
- 2 large eggs
- 1 tablespoon matcha powder
- 1 teaspoon vanilla extract

For the Topping:

- Whipped cream (optional)
- Matcha powder for dusting

Instructions:

1. Preheat your oven to 325°F (163°C). Line a square or rectangular baking pan with parchment paper leaving some overhang for easy removal.

2. In a bowl, combine almond flour, melted coconut oil, maple syrup and a pinch of salt to create the crust mixture.

3. Press the crust mixture evenly into the bottom of the prepared baking pan.

4. Bake the crust in the preheated oven for about 10 minutes or until it's lightly golden. Allow it to cool while preparing the filling.

5. In a large bowl, beat the softened cream cheese and powdered sugar until smooth.

6. Add the eggs one at a time, beating well after each addition.

7. Mix in matcha powder and vanilla extract until the filling is evenly green and well combined.

8. Pour the matcha cheesecake filling over the cooled crust and spread it evenly.

9. Bake in the oven for 25-30 minutes or until the edges are set, and the center is slightly jiggly.

10. Allow the Matcha Green Tea Cheesecake to cool completely in the pan, then refrigerate for at least 4 hours or overnight.

11. Once chilled, use the parchment paper overhang to lift the cheesecake from the pan. Cut it into bite-sized squares.

12. Optional: Pipe a small dollop of whipped cream on each cheesecake bite and dust with a sprinkle of matcha powder.

13. Serve and enjoy these delightful Matcha Green Tea Cheesecake Bites!

Coconut-Lime Chia Pudding:

Ingredients:

- 1/4 cup chia seeds
- 1 cup coconut milk (canned or homemade)
- 1 tablespoon maple syrup or agave nectar
- Zest of 1 lime
- Juice of 1 lime
- 1/2 teaspoon vanilla extract
- Shredded coconut and lime slices for garnish

Instructions:

1. In a bowl, combine chia seeds, coconut milk, maple syrup or agave nectar, lime zest, lime juice, and vanilla extract.

2. Whisk the ingredients together until well combined.

3. Let the mixture sit for a few minutes and then whisk again to prevent clumping.

4. Cover the bowl and refrigerate the Coconut-Lime Chia Pudding for at least 3 hours or overnight, allowing it to thicken.

5. Before serving, give the pudding a good stir to make sure the chia seeds are evenly distributed.

6. Spoon the chia pudding into serving glasses or bowls.

7. Optional: Garnish with shredded coconut and lime slices for added flavor and freshness.

8. Serve and enjoy.

Turmeric Golden Milk Popsicles:

Ingredients:

- 2 cups coconut milk
- 1 teaspoon ground turmeric
- 1/2 teaspoon ground ginger
- 1/4 teaspoon ground cinnamon
- 1-2 tablespoons honey or maple syrup (adjust to taste)
- 1/2 teaspoon vanilla extract
- Pinch of black pepper (enhances turmeric absorption)
- Optional: A small pinch of ground cardamom

Instructions:

1. In a saucepan, warm the coconut milk over medium heat. Add ground turmeric, ground ginger, ground cinnamon, honey or maple syrup, vanilla extract, black pepper and ground cardamom (if using).

2. Whisk the ingredients together until well combined.

3. Heat the mixture gently, but do not bring it to a boil. Allow it to simmer for 5-7 minutes, stirring occasionally.
4. Remove the saucepan from the heat and let the turmeric golden milk mixture cool to room temperature.
5. Once cooled, pour the golden milk into popsicle molds.
6. Place the molds in the freezer and let them set for about 1-2 hours.
7. After 1-2 hours, insert popsicle sticks into the semi-frozen popsicles.
8. Continue freezing the Turmeric Golden Milk Popsicles for at least 4-6 hours or until fully set.
9. Before serving, run the popsicle molds briefly under warm water to release the popsicles.
10. Enjoy these refreshing and anti-inflammatory Turmeric Golden Milk Popsicles as a unique and healthful treat!

CHAPTER 7: SMOOTHIES AND BEVERAGES TO SUPPORT HEALING

Immune Booster Smoothie:

Ingredients:

- 1 cup mixed berries (strawberries, blueberries, raspberries)
- 1 ripe banana
- 1/2 cup fresh orange juice
- 1/2 cup Greek yogurt
- 1 tablespoon honey
- 1/2 teaspoon turmeric powder
- 1/2 teaspoon ginger powder
- 1 cup spinach leaves (optional)
- 1 cup ice cubes

Instructions:

1. In a blender, combine mixed berries, ripe banana, fresh orange juice, Greek yogurt, honey, turmeric powder, ginger powder and spinach leaves (if using).
2. Add ice cubes to the blender to make the smoothie cold and refreshing.
3. Blend the ingredients until smooth and well combined.
4. Taste the smoothie and adjust sweetness or thickness by adding more honey or adjusting the amount of liquid.
5. Pour the Immune Booster Smoothie into glasses and serve immediately.
6. Optional: Garnish with fresh berries or a sprinkle of chia seeds for added texture.

Anti-Inflammatory Berry Bliss:

Ingredients:

- 1 cup mixed berries (blueberries, strawberries, raspberries)
- 1/2 cup pineapple chunks
- 1/2 cup cucumber, peeled and sliced
- 1 tablespoon chia seeds
- 1 tablespoon flaxseed meal
- 1/2 teaspoon turmeric powder
- 1/2 teaspoon ginger powder
- 1 cup coconut water or water
- Ice cubes

Instructions:

1. In a blender, combine mixed berries, pineapple chunks, cucumber slices, chia seeds, flaxseed meal, turmeric powder, ginger powder and coconut water (or water).
2. Add ice cubes to the blender for a refreshing and chilled Anti-Inflammatory Berry Bliss smoothie.
3. Blend the ingredients until smooth and well combined.
4. Taste the smoothie and adjust thickness or sweetness by adding more liquid or adjusting the amount of fruit.
5. Pour the Anti-Inflammatory Berry Bliss smoothie into glasses and serve immediately.
6. Optional: Garnish with additional chia seeds or a slice of cucumber for a decorative touch.

Detox Green Smoothie:

Ingredients:

- 1 cup kale leaves, stems removed
- 1/2 cucumber, peeled and sliced
- 1/2 green apple, cored and chopped
- 1/2 lemon, juiced
- 1 tablespoon fresh ginger, peeled and grated
- 1 tablespoon chia seeds
- 1 cup coconut water or water
- Ice cubes

Instructions:

1. In a blender, combine kale leaves, sliced cucumber, chopped green apple, lemon juice, grated fresh ginger, chia seeds and coconut water (or water).
2. Add ice cubes to the blender for a refreshing and chilled Detox Green Smoothie.
3. Blend the ingredients until smooth and well combined.
4. Taste the smoothie and adjust thickness or sweetness by adding more liquid or adjusting the amount of fruit.
5. Pour the Detox Green Smoothie into glasses and serve immediately.
6. Optional: Garnish with a slice of lemon or a few extra chia seeds for visual appeal.

Digestive Harmony Smoothie:

Ingredients:

- 1 cup pineapple chunks
- 1/2 cup papaya chunks
- 1/2 banana
- 1/2 cup Greek yogurt
- 1 tablespoon chia seeds
- 1 tablespoon fresh mint leaves
- 1/2 teaspoon ginger, grated

- 1/2 teaspoon fennel seeds
- 1 cup coconut water or water
- Ice cubes

Instructions:

1. In a blender, combine pineapple chunks, papaya chunks, banana, Greek yogurt, chia seeds, fresh mint leaves, grated ginger, fennel seeds and coconut water (or water).

2. Add ice cubes to the blender for a refreshing and chilled Digestive Harmony Smoothie.

3. Blend the ingredients until smooth and well combined.

4. Taste the smoothie and adjust thickness or sweetness by adding more liquid or adjusting the amount of fruit.

5. Pour the Digestive Harmony Smoothie into glasses and serve immediately.

6. Optional: Garnish with a sprig of fresh mint or a slice of pineapple for an extra touch.

Recovery Protein Shake:

Ingredients:

- 1 cup almond milk or any milk of your choice
- 1 scoop vanilla protein powder
- 1/2 banana, frozen
- 1 tablespoon almond butter
- 1/2 teaspoon cinnamon
- 1/2 teaspoon honey or maple syrup (optional)
- Ice cubes

Instructions:

1. In a blender, combine almond milk, vanilla protein powder, frozen banana, almond butter, cinnamon and honey or maple syrup (if using).
2. Add ice cubes to the blender for a refreshing and chilled Recovery Protein Shake.
3. Blend the ingredients until smooth and well combined.
4. Taste the protein shake and adjust sweetness or thickness by adding more honey or adjusting the amount of liquid.
5. Pour the Recovery Protein Shake into a glass and serve immediately.
6. Optional: Garnish with a sprinkle of cinnamon or a few sliced almonds for added texture.

Hydrating Coconut Watermelon Refresher:

Ingredients:

- 2 cups watermelon, diced
- 1 cup coconut water
- Juice of 1 lime
- 1 tablespoon fresh mint leaves, chopped
- 1 tablespoon honey or agave syrup (optional)
- Ice cubes

Instructions:

1. In a blender, combine diced watermelon, coconut water, lime juice, chopped mint leaves and honey or agave syrup (if using).
2. Add ice cubes to the blender for a refreshing and hydrating Coconut Watermelon Refresher.
3. Blend the ingredients until smooth and well combined.
4. Taste the refresher and adjust sweetness or thickness by adding more honey or adjusting the amount of watermelon.
5. Pour the Coconut Watermelon Refresher into glasses and serve immediately.
6. Optional: Garnish with a sprig of fresh mint or a slice of watermelon for an extra touch.

Cleansing Citrus Delight:

Ingredients:

- 1 grapefruit, peeled and segmented
- 2 oranges, peeled and segmented
- 1 lemon, juiced
- 1 tablespoon fresh ginger, grated
- 1 tablespoon honey or agave syrup (optional)
- 1 cup cold water
- Ice cubes

Instructions:

1. In a blender, combine grapefruit segments, orange segments, lemon juice, grated ginger, honey or agave syrup (if using) and cold water.
2. Add ice cubes to the blender for a refreshing and cleansing Citrus Delight.
3. Blend the ingredients until smooth and well combined.
4. Taste the drink and adjust sweetness or thickness by adding more honey or adjusting the amount of citrus.
5. Pour the Cleansing Citrus Delight into glasses and serve immediately.
6. Optional: Garnish with a twist of citrus peel or a sprig of fresh mint for an extra burst of flavor.

Berries and Beet Energizer:

Ingredients:

- 1/2 cup blueberries
- 1/2 cup strawberries, hulled and halved
- 1 small beet, peeled and diced
- 1 tablespoon chia seeds
- 1 tablespoon fresh mint leaves, chopped
- 1 tablespoon honey or agave syrup (optional)
- 1 cup cold water

- Ice cubes

Instructions:

1. In a blender, combine blueberries, strawberries, diced beet, chia seeds, chopped mint leaves, honey or agave syrup (if using) and cold water.
2. Add ice cubes to the blender for a refreshing and energizing Berries and Beet Energizer.
3. Blend the ingredients until smooth and well combined.
4. Taste the drink and adjust sweetness or thickness by adding more honey or adjusting the amount of berries.
5. Pour the Berries and Beet Energizer into glasses and serve immediately.
6. Optional: Garnish with a few whole berries or a sprig of fresh mint for visual appeal.

Healing Turmeric Mango Lassi:

Ingredients:

- 1 cup ripe mango, diced
- 1 cup plain yogurt (or coconut yogurt for a dairy-free option)
- 1/2 cup cold water
- 1/2 teaspoon ground turmeric
- 1/2 teaspoon ground cardamom
- 1 tablespoon honey or agave syrup (adjust to taste)
- Pinch of black pepper (enhances turmeric absorption)
- Ice cubes

Instructions:

1. In a blender, combine diced mango, plain yogurt, cold water, ground turmeric, ground cardamom, honey or agave syrup and a pinch of black pepper.
2. Add ice cubes to the blender for a cooling and healing Turmeric Mango Lassi.
3. Blend the ingredients until smooth and well combined.

4. Taste the lassi and adjust sweetness or thickness by adding more honey or adjusting the amount of mango.

5. Pour the Healing Turmeric Mango Lassi into glasses and serve immediately.

6. Optional: Garnish with a sprinkle of ground turmeric or a slice of fresh mango for an extra touch.

Probiotic Pineapple Green Smoothie:

Ingredients:

- 1 cup fresh pineapple chunks
- 1 cup spinach leaves
- 1/2 cup cucumber, peeled and sliced
- 1/2 banana
- 1 cup coconut water or water
- 1/2 cup Greek yogurt (or dairy-free yogurt for a vegan option)
- 1 tablespoon chia seeds
- 1 tablespoon honey or agave syrup (optional)
- Ice cubes

Instructions:

1. In a blender, combine fresh pineapple chunks, spinach leaves, sliced cucumber, banana, coconut water (or water) Greek yogurt, chia seeds and honey or agave syrup (if using).

2. Add ice cubes to the blender for a refreshing and probiotic-rich Pineapple Green Smoothie.

3. Blend the ingredients until smooth and well combined.

4. Taste the smoothie and adjust sweetness or thickness by adding more honey or adjusting the amount of pineapple.

5. Pour the Probiotic Pineapple Green Smoothie into glasses and serve immediately.

6. Optional: Garnish with a slice of pineapple or a sprinkle of chia seeds for an extra touch.

Calming Chamomile Banana Smoothie:

Ingredients:

- 1 banana
- 1/2 cup chamomile tea, cooled
- 1/2 cup Greek yogurt (or dairy-free yogurt for a vegan option)
- 1 tablespoon almond butter
- 1 teaspoon honey or agave syrup (optional)
- 1/2 teaspoon vanilla extract
- Ice cubes

Instructions:

1. Brew chamomile tea and allow it to cool to room temperature.
2. In a blender, combine a ripe banana, cooled chamomile tea, Greek yogurt (or dairy-free yogurt), almond butter, honey or agave syrup (if using), vanilla extract and ice cubes.
3. Blend the ingredients until smooth and well combined.
4. Taste the smoothie and adjust sweetness or thickness by adding more honey or adjusting the amount of banana.
5. Pour the Calming Chamomile Banana Smoothie into glasses and serve immediately.
6. Optional: Garnish with a drizzle of honey or a sprinkle of chamomile flowers for a calming visual touch.

Cherry Almond Antioxidant Smoothie:

Ingredients:

- 1 cup frozen cherries
- 1/2 cup almond milk
- 1/2 cup Greek yogurt (or dairy-free yogurt for a vegan option)
- 1 tablespoon almond butter
- 1 tablespoon chia seeds

- 1 tablespoon honey or agave syrup (optional)
- 1/4 teaspoon almond extract
- Ice cubes

Instructions:

1. In a blender, combine frozen cherries, almond milk, Greek yogurt (or dairy-free yogurt), almond butter, chia seeds, honey or agave syrup (if using), almond extract and ice cubes.
2. Blend the ingredients until smooth and well combined.
3. Taste the smoothie and adjust sweetness or thickness by adding more honey or adjusting the amount of cherries.
4. Pour the Cherry Almond Antioxidant Smoothie into glasses and serve immediately.
5. Optional: Garnish with a few whole cherries or a sprinkle of sliced almonds for added texture.

Post-Workout Coconut Berry Refuel:

Ingredients:

- 1/2 cup mixed berries (blueberries, strawberries, raspberries)
- 1/2 banana
- 1/2 cup coconut water
- 1/2 cup Greek yogurt (or dairy-free yogurt for a vegan option)
- 1 tablespoon chia seeds
- 1 tablespoon almond butter
- 1 teaspoon honey or agave syrup (optional)
- Ice cubes

Instructions:

1. In a blender, combine mixed berries, banana, coconut water, Greek yogurt (or dairy-free yogurt) chia seeds, almond butter, honey or agave syrup (if using), and ice cubes.

2. Blend the ingredients until smooth and well combined.

3. Taste the smoothie and adjust sweetness or thickness by adding more honey or adjusting the amount of berries.

4. Pour the Post-Workout Coconut Berry Refuel smoothie into glasses and serve immediately.

5. Optional: Garnish with a drizzle of honey or a few extra berries for a burst of color.

Gut-Healing Aloe Vera Citrus Smoothie:

Ingredients:

- 1 cup aloe vera juice (pure and edible)
- 1/2 cup orange juice
- 1/2 cup pineapple chunks
- 1/2 banana
- 1 tablespoon chia seeds
- 1 tablespoon honey or agave syrup (optional)
- Ice cubes

Instructions:

1. In a blender, combine aloe vera juice, orange juice, pineapple chunks, banana, chia seeds, honey or agave syrup (if using) and ice cubes.

2. Blend the ingredients until smooth and well combined.

3. Taste the smoothie and adjust sweetness or thickness by adding more honey or adjusting the amount of pineapple.

4. Pour the Gut-Healing Aloe Vera Citrus Smoothie into glasses and serve immediately.

5. Optional: Garnish with a slice of orange or a sprinkle of chia seeds for visual appeal.

Elderberry Immunity Elixir:

Ingredients:

- 1 cup elderberry juice or elderberry syrup
- 1/2 lemon, juiced
- 1 tablespoon raw honey
- 1-inch piece of fresh ginger, grated
- 1/2 teaspoon ground cinnamon
- 1/4 teaspoon ground cloves
- 1 cup hot water

Instructions:

1. In a mug, combine elderberry juice or syrup, freshly squeezed lemon juice, raw honey, grated ginger, ground cinnamon and ground cloves.
2. Pour hot water over the ingredients in the mug.
3. Stir the mixture well until the honey is fully dissolved.
4. Let the Elderberry Immunity Elixir steep for a few minutes to allow the flavors to meld and the elixir to cool slightly.
5. Optional: Strain the elixir to remove grated ginger if desired.
6. Sip on this comforting and immune-boosting elixir while it's warm.
7. Enjoy this Elderberry Immunity Elixir as a soothing and healthful beverage.

Beverages to Support Healing

Turmeric Golden Milk Latte:

Ingredients:

- 1 cup milk (dairy or plant-based)
- 1/2 teaspoon ground turmeric
- 1/4 teaspoon ground cinnamon
- 1/4 teaspoon ground ginger
- Pinch of black pepper (enhances turmeric absorption)

* 1 tablespoon honey or maple syrup (adjust to taste)
* 1/2 teaspoon vanilla extract

Instructions:

1. In a small saucepan, heat the milk over medium heat.
2. Add ground turmeric, ground cinnamon, ground ginger, black pepper, honey or maple syrup and vanilla extract to the milk.
3. Whisk the mixture continuously while heating to ensure the spices are well incorporated and the milk is warmed through.
4. Continue heating the Turmeric Golden Milk Latte until it's hot but not boiling.
5. Remove the saucepan from the heat.
6. Optional: Use a frother to create a frothy texture on top of the latte.
7. Pour the Turmeric Golden Milk Latte into a mug.
8. Optional: Sprinkle a little extra ground cinnamon on top for garnish.
9. Enjoy this comforting and anti-inflammatory drink!

Herbal Tea Blend for Relaxation:

Ingredients:

* 1 tablespoon dried chamomile flowers
* 1 tablespoon dried lavender buds
* 1 tablespoon dried lemon balm leaves
* 1 tablespoon dried passion flower
* 1 teaspoon dried peppermint leaves
* Optional: 1 teaspoon dried rose petals

Instructions:

1. In a bowl, combine dried chamomile flowers, lavender buds, lemon balm leaves, passionflower, peppermint leaves and if desired, dried rose petals.
2. Mix the herbs together thoroughly to create a well-blended herbal tea blend.
3. To make a cup of herbal tea, use 1-2 teaspoons of the herbal tea blend per 8 ounces of hot water.

4. Place the herbal tea blend in a tea infuser or directly into a teapot.

5. Pour hot water over the herbal tea blend.

6. Let the tea steep for about 5-7 minutes to allow the herbs to release their flavors and aromas.

7. Strain the tea if necessary or simply remove the tea infuser.

8. Optional: Sweeten the tea with honey or another sweetener if desired.

9. Pour the Herbal Tea Blend for Relaxation into a cup and enjoy this soothing and calming beverage.

Ginger Lemon Detox Water:

Ingredients:

- 1 inch piece of fresh ginger, thinly sliced
- 1 lemon, thinly sliced
- 1-2 tablespoons apple cider vinegar (optional)
- 1-2 teaspoons honey or agave syrup (optional)
- 4 cups water (filtered or still water)
- Ice cubes (optional)

Instructions:

1. In a large pitcher, combine thinly sliced fresh ginger and lemon slices.

2. If desired, add apple cider vinegar for an extra detox boost.

3. Optionally, add honey or agave syrup for a touch of sweetness.

4. Pour 4 cups of water over the ginger and lemon slices.

5. Stir the ingredients well to ensure they are evenly distributed.

6. Refrigerate the Ginger Lemon Detox Water for at least 2-4 hours, allowing the flavors to infuse.

7. Before serving, you can add ice cubes for a refreshing chill.

8. Pour the detox water into glasses, ensuring that some ginger and lemon slices are included in each serving.

9. Enjoy this invigorating and cleansing Ginger Lemon Detox Water as a hydrating beverage.

Minty Cucumber Infused Water:

Ingredients:

- 1/2 cucumber, thinly sliced
- 1/2 lemon, thinly sliced
- Fresh mint leaves
- 4 cups water (filtered or still water)
- Ice cubes (optional)

Instructions:

1. In a large pitcher, combine thinly sliced cucumber and lemon slices.
2. Add fresh mint leaves to the pitcher. Use as much as you prefer depending on how minty you want your infused water.
3. Pour 4 cups of water over the cucumber, lemon, and mint in the pitcher.
4. Stir the ingredients gently to distribute the flavors.
5. Refrigerate the Minty Cucumber Infused Water for at least 2-4 hours, allowing the flavors to infuse.
6. Before serving, you can add ice cubes for a refreshing chill.
7. Pour the infused water into glasses, ensuring that some cucumber, lemon and mint are included in each serving.
8. Enjoy this crisp and minty infused water as a hydrating and flavorful beverage.

Green Tea with Matcha Boost:

Ingredients:

- 1 green tea bag
- 1/2 teaspoon matcha powder
- 1 cup hot water (not boiling)
- Honey or sweetener of choice (optional)

Instructions:

1. Place the green tea bag in a cup.
2. In a separate bowl, whisk matcha powder with a small amount of hot water until it forms a smooth paste.
3. Heat the remaining water until it's hot but not boiling.
4. Pour the hot water over the green tea bag in the cup.
5. Add the matcha paste to the cup with the green tea.
6. Optional: Sweeten the tea with honey or your preferred sweetener, stirring to dissolve.
7. Allow the Green Tea with Matcha Boost to steep for 2-3 minutes.
8. Remove the green tea bag and stir the matcha mixture thoroughly.
9. Enjoy this invigorating Green Tea with Matcha Boost as a soothing and energizing drink.

Spiced Apple Cider Vinegar Tonic:

Ingredients:

- 1 cup water
- 1 tablespoon apple cider vinegar (with the mother)
- 1 tablespoon lemon juice
- 1 tablespoon honey or maple syrup
- 1/2 teaspoon ground cinnamon
- 1/4 teaspoon ground turmeric
- Pinch of cayenne pepper (optional)

Instructions:

1. Heat the water until warm but not boiling.
2. In a mug, combine warm water, apple cider vinegar, lemon juice, honey or maple syrup, ground cinnamon, ground turmeric and a pinch of cayenne pepper if you like it spicy.
3. Stir the Spiced Apple Cider Vinegar Tonic until all ingredients are well mixed.

4. Allow the tonic to cool to a comfortable temperature for drinking.

5. Sip and enjoy the warm and spiced flavors of this tonic.

Blueberry Lavender Lemonade:

Ingredients:

- 1 cup blueberries (fresh or frozen)
- 1/2 cup dried culinary lavender
- 1 cup hot water
- 1 cup fresh lemon juice (about 4-5 lemons)
- 1/2 cup honey or agave syrup (adjust to taste)
- 4 cups cold water
- Ice cubes
- Fresh lavender sprigs and blueberries for garnish (optional)

Instructions:

1. In a heatproof bowl, combine dried culinary lavender with hot water. Let it steep for about 10-15 minutes to infuse the lavender flavor.

2. Strain the lavender-infused water to remove the lavender buds, leaving behind the lavender-infused liquid.

3. In a blender, combine blueberries and fresh lemon juice. Blend until smooth.

4. In a large pitcher, combine the blueberry-lemon mixture, lavender-infused water, honey or agave syrup, and cold water. Stir well to mix.

5. Taste the Blueberry Lavender Lemonade and adjust sweetness or tartness by adding more honey or lemon juice as needed.

6. Refrigerate the lemonade for at least 1-2 hours to allow the flavors to meld.

7. Before serving, add ice cubes to the pitcher for a refreshing chill.

8. Optional: Garnish individual glasses with fresh lavender sprigs and a few whole blueberries.

9. Pour the Blueberry Lavender Lemonade into glasses and enjoy this uniquely flavored and refreshing beverage.

Pomegranate Hibiscus Iced Tea:

Ingredients:

- 2 hibiscus tea bags
- 1/2 cup dried hibiscus petals
- 4 cups hot water
- 1/2 cup pomegranate juice
- 1/4 cup honey or agave syrup (adjust to taste)
- Ice cubes
- Pomegranate arils and mint leaves for garnish (optional)

Instructions:

1. In a heatproof pitcher, combine hibiscus tea bags and dried hibiscus petals.
2. Pour hot water over the tea bags and hibiscus petals.
3. Let the mixture steep for about 10-15 minutes, allowing the vibrant hibiscus flavor to infuse into the water.
4. Remove the tea bags and strain out the hibiscus petals, leaving behind the hibiscus-infused liquid.
5. Stir in pomegranate juice and honey or agave syrup until well combined.
6. Refrigerate the Pomegranate Hibiscus Iced Tea for at least 1-2 hours to chill and allow the flavors to meld.
7. Before serving, add ice cubes to the pitcher for a refreshing chill.
8. Optionally, garnish individual glasses with pomegranate arils and mint leaves.
9. Pour the iced tea into glasses and enjoy the delightful combination of hibiscus and pomegranate.

Rosemary Citrus Sparkler:

Ingredients:

- 1 sprig fresh rosemary
- 1/2 lemon, juiced
- 1/2 orange, juiced

- 1 tablespoon honey or agave syrup

- 1 cup sparkling water

- Ice cubes

- Lemon or orange slices for garnish (optional)

Instructions:

1. In a glass, muddle the fresh rosemary to release its aromatic oils.

2. Add the freshly squeezed lemon juice, orange juice and honey or agave syrup to the glass.

3. Stir the ingredients well to dissolve the honey or agave syrup.

4. Add ice cubes to the glass for a refreshing chill.

5. Pour sparkling water over the mixture, gently stirring to combine.

6. Optionally, garnish the Rosemary Citrus Sparkler with lemon or orange slices.

7. Enjoy this herbal and citrusy sparkling beverage as a refreshing and flavorful drink.

Protein-Packed Almond Milkshake:

Ingredients:

- 1 cup almond milk

- 1 banana, frozen

- 1/4 cup almonds, preferably soaked and peeled

- 1 tablespoon almond butter

- 1 scoop vanilla protein powder

- 1/2 teaspoon cinnamon

- 1/2 teaspoon vanilla extract

- Ice cubes (optional)

- Sweetener of choice, if desired (optional)

Instructions:

1. In a blender, combine almond milk, frozen banana, almonds, almond butter, vanilla protein powder, cinnamon and vanilla extract.

2. If you prefer a colder shake, add ice cubes to the blender.

3. Optionally, sweeten the shake with your preferred sweetener, adjusting to taste.

4. Blend the ingredients until smooth and well combined.

5. Taste the shake and adjust sweetness or thickness by adding more sweetener or adjusting the amount of almond milk.

6. Pour the Protein-Packed Almond Milkshake into a glass.

7. Optional: Garnish with a sprinkle of cinnamon or a few chopped almonds for added texture.

Cranberry Kombucha Cooler:

Ingredients:

- 1 cup cranberry juice (unsweetened)
- 1 cup kombucha (plain or flavored, depending on preference)
- 1 tablespoon honey or agave syrup (adjust to taste)
- 1/2 lemon, juiced
- Ice cubes
- Fresh cranberries and mint leaves for garnish (optional)

Instructions:

1. In a pitcher, combine cranberry juice, kombucha, honey or agave syrup and freshly squeezed lemon juice.

2. Stir the ingredients well to ensure they are thoroughly mixed.

3. Taste the mixture and adjust sweetness by adding more honey or agave syrup if needed.

4. Refrigerate the Cranberry Kombucha Cooler for at least 1-2 hours to chill and allow the flavors to meld.

5. Before serving, add ice cubes to the pitcher for a refreshing chill.

6. Optionally, garnish individual glasses with fresh cranberries and mint leaves.

7. Pour the cooler into glasses and enjoy the tangy and effervescent combination of cranberry and kombucha.

Soothing Lavender Almond Latte:

Ingredients:

- 1 cup almond milk
- 1/2 teaspoon dried culinary lavender
- 1 tablespoon almond butter
- 1 teaspoon honey or agave syrup (adjust to taste)
- 1/2 teaspoon vanilla extract
- 1 shot of espresso or 1/2 cup strong brewed coffee
- Lavender buds for garnish (optional)

Instructions:

1. In a small saucepan, heat almond milk over medium heat until it's warm but not boiling.
2. Place dried culinary lavender in a tea infuser or a small cloth bag and add it to the almond milk. Let it steep for about 5 minutes to infuse the lavender flavor.
3. Remove the lavender-infused almond milk from the heat and discard the lavender.
4. In a blender, combine the lavender-infused almond milk, almond butter, honey or agave syrup and vanilla extract. Blend until frothy.
5. Prepare a shot of espresso or 1/2 cup strong brewed coffee.
6. Pour the espresso or coffee into a mug.
7. Pour the lavender almond milk mixture over the espresso or coffee in the mug.
8. Optional: Garnish with a sprinkle of lavender buds for a visual touch.
9. Stir the Soothing Lavender Almond Latte gently and enjoy this calming and aromatic beverage.

Coconut Pineapple Electrolyte Refresher:

Ingredients:

- 1 cup coconut water

- 1/2 cup pineapple juice
- 1/4 cup freshly squeezed lime juice
- 1-2 tablespoons honey or agave syrup (adjust to taste)
- Pinch of sea salt
- Ice cubes
- Pineapple slices and mint leaves for garnish (optional)

Instructions:

1. In a pitcher, combine coconut water, pineapple juice, freshly squeezed lime juice, honey or agave syrup and a pinch of sea salt.
2. Stir the ingredients well to dissolve the sweetener and sea salt.
3. Taste the Coconut Pineapple Electrolyte Refresher and adjust sweetness or saltiness as needed.
4. Refrigerate the refresher for at least 1-2 hours to chill and allow the flavors to meld.
5. Before serving, add ice cubes to the pitcher for a refreshing chill.
6. Optionally, garnish individual glasses with pineapple slices and mint leaves.
7. Pour the refresher into glasses and enjoy this hydrating and tropical electrolyte boost.

Ginseng Green Tea Elixir:

Ingredients:

- 1 cup green tea, brewed and cooled
- 1 teaspoon ginseng powder
- 1 tablespoon honey or agave syrup (adjust to taste)
- 1/2 lemon, juiced
- Ice cubes
- Lemon slices for garnish (optional)

Instructions:

1. Brew green tea according to package instructions and allow it to cool to room temperature.
2. In a glass, combine the cooled green tea, ginseng powder, honey or agave syrup and freshly squeezed lemon juice.
3. Stir the ingredients well to ensure they are thoroughly mixed.
4. Taste the Ginseng Green Tea Elixir and adjust sweetness or tartness by adding more honey or lemon juice as needed.
5. Add ice cubes to the glass for a refreshing chill.
6. Optionally, garnish with lemon slices for a visual touch.
7. Stir again before serving, and enjoy this invigorating and healthful elixir.

Cinnamon Vanilla Date Milk:

Ingredients:

- 1 cup almond milk (or any milk of choice)
- 2-3 Medjool dates, pitted
- 1/2 teaspoon ground cinnamon
- 1/2 teaspoon vanilla extract
- Pinch of sea salt
- Ice cubes (optional)

Instructions:

1. In a blender, combine almond milk, pitted Medjool dates, ground cinnamon, vanilla extract and a pinch of sea salt.
2. Blend the ingredients until the dates are fully incorporated and the mixture becomes smooth and creamy.
3. Taste the Cinnamon Vanilla Date Milk and adjust sweetness or cinnamon to your liking.

4. If desired, add ice cubes to the blender and blend again for a chilled version.

5. Pour the Cinnamon Vanilla Date Milk into a glass.

6. Optional: Sprinkle a little extra ground cinnamon on top for garnish.

7. Enjoy this naturally sweetened and flavorful date milk as a delicious and nourishing beverage.

Roasted Tomato Basil Soup:

Ingredients:

- 1.5 lbs (about 680g) tomatoes, halved
- 1 onion, roughly chopped
- 4 cloves garlic, peeled
- 2 tablespoons olive oil
- Salt and pepper to taste
- 1 teaspoon dried oregano
- 1 teaspoon dried thyme
- 1/2 teaspoon red pepper flakes (optional for a hint of heat)
- 4 cups vegetable or chicken broth
- 1/2 cup fresh basil leaves, plus extra for garnish
- 1/2 cup heavy cream (optional for added richness)
- Grated Parmesan cheese for serving (optional)

Instructions:

1. Preheat your oven to 400°F (200°C).
2. Place the halved tomatoes, chopped onion and peeled garlic cloves on a baking sheet.
3. Drizzle olive oil over the tomatoes, onion and garlic. Sprinkle with salt, pepper, dried oregano, dried thyme and red pepper flakes if using.
4. Toss everything on the baking sheet to ensure the vegetables are well coated with the oil and seasoning.
5. Roast in the preheated oven for about 30-40 minutes or until the tomatoes are caramelized and the onions are soft and golden.
6. Transfer the roasted vegetables to a blender. Add fresh basil leaves.
7. Pour in the vegetable or chicken broth.

8. Blend until smooth. You may need to do this in batches depending on the size of your blender.

9. Pour the blended mixture into a pot and bring to a simmer over medium heat.

10. Stir in the heavy cream if using and let it simmer for an additional 5-10 minutes.

11. Taste and adjust seasoning if needed.

12. Serve the Roasted Tomato Basil Soup hot, garnished with additional fresh basil leaves and a sprinkle of grated Parmesan cheese if desired.

Chicken and Vegetable Noodle Soup:

Ingredients:

- 1 tablespoon olive oil
- 1 onion, diced
- 2 carrots, sliced
- 2 celery stalks, sliced
- 2 cloves garlic, minced
- 1 teaspoon dried thyme
- 1 teaspoon dried oregano
- 8 cups chicken broth
- 2 boneless, skinless chicken breasts, cooked and shredded
- 2 cups egg noodles
- Salt and pepper to taste
- Fresh parsley, chopped, for garnish (optional)
- Lemon wedges for serving (optional)

Instructions:

1. In a large pot, heat olive oil over medium heat. Add diced onion, sliced carrots and sliced celery. Cook until the vegetables begin to soften about 5 minutes.

2. Add minced garlic, dried thyme, and dried oregano to the pot. Cook for an additional 1-2 minutes, stirring frequently to release the flavors.

3. Pour in the chicken broth and bring the mixture to a simmer.

4. Add the shredded chicken to the pot.

5. Stir in the egg noodles and let the soup simmer until the noodles are cooked usually about 8-10 minutes. Check the package instructions for the recommended cooking time.

6. Season the soup with salt and pepper to taste. Adjust the seasoning as needed.

7. Ladle the Chicken and Vegetable Noodle Soup into bowls.

8. Garnish with chopped fresh parsley if desired.

9. Serve the soup hot with optional lemon wedges on the side for an extra burst of flavor.

Creamy Butternut Squash Soup:

Ingredients:

- 1 medium-sized butternut squash, peeled, seeded and diced
- 1 onion, chopped
- 2 carrots, peeled and chopped
- 2 cloves garlic, minced
- 1 apple, peeled, cored, and chopped
- 4 cups vegetable or chicken broth
- 1 teaspoon ground cinnamon
- 1/2 teaspoon ground nutmeg
- Salt and pepper to taste
- 2 tablespoons olive oil
- 1 cup coconut milk or heavy cream
- Toasted pumpkin seeds for garnish (optional)
- Fresh thyme leaves for garnish (optional)

Instructions:

1. In a large pot, heat the olive oil over medium heat. Add the chopped onion, carrots and garlic. Saute until the vegetables are softened about 5-7 minutes.

2. Add the diced butternut squash and apple to the pot. Continue to cook for an additional 5 minutes stirring occasionally.

3. Pour in the vegetable or chicken broth, ensuring it covers the vegetables. Bring the mixture to a simmer and cook until the butternut squash is tender about 20-25 minutes.

4. Use an immersion blender to carefully blend the soup until smooth. Alternatively, transfer the soup in batches to a blender and blend until smooth then return to the pot.

5. Season the soup with ground cinnamon, ground nutmeg, salt and pepper. Stir well to combine.

6. Stir in the coconut milk or heavy cream, and let the soup simmer for an additional 5-10 minutes.

7. Taste and adjust seasoning as needed.

8. Ladle the Creamy Butternut Squash Soup into bowls.

9. Garnish with toasted pumpkin seeds and fresh thyme leaves if desired.

10. Serve the soup hot and enjoy the rich velvety flavors!

Lentil and Vegetable Soup:

Ingredients:

- 1 cup dry green or brown lentils, rinsed and drained
- 1 onion, diced
- 2 carrots, peeled and diced
- 2 celery stalks, diced
- 3 cloves garlic, minced
- 1 can (14 oz) diced tomatoes
- 6 cups vegetable broth
- 1 teaspoon ground cumin
- 1 teaspoon ground coriander
- 1 teaspoon smoked paprika

- 1 bay leaf
- Salt and pepper to taste
- 2 tablespoons olive oil
- Fresh parsley, chopped, for garnish (optional)
- Lemon wedges for serving (optional)

Instructions:

1. In a large pot, heat olive oil over medium heat. Add diced onion, carrots, and celery. Cook until the vegetables are softened about 5-7 minutes.
2. Add minced garlic and cook for an additional 1-2 minutes stirring frequently.
3. Pour in the vegetable broth and add the rinsed lentils, diced tomatoes (with their juices), ground cumin, ground coriander, smoked paprika, bay leaf, salt and pepper.
4. Bring the soup to a boil, then reduce the heat to low, cover and simmer for about 25-30 minutes or until the lentils are tender.
5. Taste the Lentil and Vegetable Soup and adjust the seasoning if needed.
6. Remove the bay leaf and discard it.
7. Ladle the soup into bowls.
8. Garnish with chopped fresh parsley if desired.
9. Serve the soup hot with optional lemon wedges on the side for a burst of citrus flavor.

Minestrone Soup:

Ingredients:

- 2 tablespoons olive oil
- 1 onion, diced
- 2 carrots, peeled and diced
- 2 celery stalks, diced
- 3 cloves garlic, minced
- 1 zucchini, diced

- 1 cup green beans, trimmed and cut into bite-sized pieces
- 1 can (14 oz) diced tomatoes
- 1 can (15 oz) kidney beans, drained and rinsed
- 6 cups vegetable broth
- 1 teaspoon dried oregano
- 1 teaspoon dried basil
- 1 teaspoon dried thyme
- 1/2 cup small pasta (e.g. ditalini or small shells)
- Salt and pepper to taste
- 2 cups fresh spinach or kale, chopped
- Grated Parmesan cheese for serving (optional)

Instructions:

1. In a large pot, heat olive oil over medium heat. Add diced onion, carrots, and celery. Cook until the vegetables are softened about 5-7 minutes.
2. Add minced garlic and cook for an additional 1-2 minutes stirring frequently.
3. Stir in diced zucchini, green beans, diced tomatoes, kidney beans, vegetable broth, dried oregano, dried basil and dried thyme.
4. Bring the soup to a boil, then reduce the heat to low, cover and simmer for about 15-20 minutes.
5. Add the small pasta to the pot and continue to simmer until the pasta is cooked about 10 minutes.
6. Season the Minestrone Soup with salt and pepper to taste.
7. Stir in chopped spinach or kale and cook until wilted about 2-3 minutes.
8. Taste and adjust the seasoning if needed.
9. Ladle the soup into bowls.
10. Optionally, sprinkle with grated Parmesan cheese before serving.
11. Serve the Minestrone Soup hot and enjoy this classic Italian vegetable soup!

Mushroom Barley Soup:

Ingredients:

- 1 cup pearl barley, rinsed and drained
- 2 tablespoons olive oil
- 1 onion, finely chopped
- 2 carrots, peeled and diced
- 2 celery stalks, diced
- 3 cloves garlic, minced
- 8 oz (about 227g) mushrooms, sliced (any variety you prefer)
- 6 cups vegetable or beef broth
- 1 teaspoon dried thyme
- 1 bay leaf
- Salt and pepper to taste
- Fresh parsley, chopped, for garnish (optional)

Instructions:

1. In a medium pot, bring 4 cups of water to a boil. Add the rinsed barley, reduce heat to low, cover, and simmer for about 30-40 minutes or until the barley is tender. Drain any excess water.
2. In a large pot, heat olive oil over medium heat. Add chopped onion, diced carrots, and diced celery. Cook until the vegetables are softened about 5-7 minutes.
3. Add minced garlic and sliced mushrooms to the pot. Cook for an additional 3-5 minutes stirring frequently.
4. Pour in the vegetable or beef broth, add cooked barley, dried thyme, bay leaf, salt and pepper.
5. Bring the Mushroom Barley Soup to a boil, then reduce the heat to low, cover and simmer for about 20-25 minutes to allow the flavors to meld.
6. Taste the soup and adjust the seasoning if needed.
7. Remove the bay leaf and discard it.
8. Ladle the soup into bowls.

9. Optionally, garnish with chopped fresh parsley.

10. Serve the Mushroom Barley Soup hot and enjoy the hearty and comforting flavors!

Thai Coconut Curry Soup:

Ingredients:

- 1 tablespoon vegetable oil
- 1 onion, finely chopped
- 2 cloves garlic, minced
- 1 tablespoon red curry paste
- 1 can (14 oz) coconut milk
- 4 cups vegetable or chicken broth
- 1 tablespoon soy sauce
- 1 tablespoon brown sugar
- 1 tablespoon fresh ginger, grated
- 2 carrots, julienned
- 1 red bell pepper, thinly sliced
- 1 cup broccoli florets
- 8 oz (about 227g) firm tofu, cubed
- 1 tablespoon lime juice
- Salt and pepper to taste
- Fresh cilantro and sliced green onions for garnish
- Cooked rice or rice noodles for serving (optional)

Instructions:

1. In a large pot, heat vegetable oil over medium heat. Add chopped onion and cook until softened about 3-5 minutes.

2. Add minced garlic and red curry paste to the pot. Stir and cook for an additional 1-2 minutes.

3. Pour in the coconut milk, vegetable or chicken broth, soy sauce, brown sugar and grated ginger. Bring the mixture to a simmer.

4. Add julienned carrots, sliced red bell pepper, broccoli florets, and cubed tofu to the pot. Simmer for about 10-15 minutes or until the vegetables are tender.

5. Stir in lime juice and season the Thai Coconut Curry Soup with salt and pepper to taste.

6. Taste and adjust the flavors by adding more lime juice, soy sauce or brown sugar if needed.

7. Ladle the soup into bowls.

8. Optionally, serve the soup over cooked rice or rice noodles.

9. Garnish with fresh cilantro and sliced green onions.

10. Serve the Thai Coconut Curry Soup hot and enjoy the rich and aromatic flavors!

Spinach and White Bean Soup:

Ingredients:

- 1 tablespoon olive oil
- 1 onion, diced
- 2 carrots, peeled and diced
- 2 celery stalks, diced
- 3 cloves garlic, minced
- 1 teaspoon dried thyme
- 2 cans (15 oz each) white beans (cannellini or Great Northern), drained and rinsed
- 6 cups vegetable or chicken broth
- 4 cups fresh spinach, chopped
- 1 teaspoon lemon zest
- Salt and pepper to taste
- Grated Parmesan cheese for serving (optional)

Instructions:

1. In a large pot, heat olive oil over medium heat. Add diced onion, carrots, and celery. Cook until the vegetables are softened about 5-7 minutes.
2. Add minced garlic and dried thyme to the pot. Cook for an additional 1-2 minutes stirring frequently.
3. Pour in the vegetable or chicken broth and add the drained white beans. Bring the mixture to a simmer.
4. Simmer for about 15-20 minutes to allow the flavors to meld.
5. Stir in the chopped fresh spinach and cook until wilted, about 2-3 minutes.
6. Add lemon zest to the pot and season the Spinach and White Bean Soup with salt and pepper to taste.
7. Taste and adjust the seasoning if needed.
8. Ladle the soup into bowls.
9. Optionally, sprinkle with grated Parmesan cheese before serving.
10. Serve the Spinach and White Bean Soup hot and enjoy this nutritious and flavorful dish!

Turmeric Carrot Ginger Soup:

Ingredients:

- 1 tablespoon coconut oil or olive oil
- 1 onion, chopped
- 2 pounds (about 907g) carrots, peeled and chopped
- 3 cloves garlic, minced
- 1 tablespoon fresh ginger, grated
- 1 teaspoon ground turmeric
- 6 cups vegetable broth
- 1 can (14 oz) coconut milk
- Salt and pepper to taste
- Pinch of cayenne pepper (optional for heat)
- Fresh cilantro or parsley, chopped, for garnish

- Toasted pumpkin seeds for garnish (optional)

Instructions:

1. In a large pot, heat coconut oil or olive oil over medium heat. Add chopped onion and cook until softened, about 5-7 minutes.
2. Add chopped carrots, minced garlic, grated ginger, and ground turmeric to the pot. Cook for an additional 3-5 minutes stirring frequently.
3. Pour in the vegetable broth and bring the mixture to a simmer. Cook until the carrots are tender about 15-20 minutes.
4. Use an immersion blender to carefully blend the soup until smooth. Alternatively, transfer the soup in batches to a blender and blend until smooth then return to the pot.
5. Stir in the coconut milk and season the Turmeric Carrot Ginger Soup with salt, pepper and cayenne pepper if using.
6. Simmer for an additional 5-10 minutes to heat through and allow the flavors to meld.
7. Taste and adjust the seasoning if needed.
8. Ladle the soup into bowls.
9. Optionally, garnish with chopped fresh cilantro or parsley and toasted pumpkin seeds.
10. Serve the Turmeric Carrot Ginger Soup hot and enjoy the vibrant and comforting flavors!

Vegetarian Borscht:

Ingredients:

- 2 tablespoons olive oil
- 1 onion, finely chopped
- 2 carrots, peeled and shredded
- 2 beets, peeled and shredded
- 2 potatoes, peeled and diced

- 1 small cabbage, shredded
- 3 cloves garlic, minced
- 1 can (14 oz) diced tomatoes
- 6 cups vegetable broth
- 2 bay leaves
- 1 teaspoon dried dill
- 1 tablespoon apple cider vinegar
- Salt and pepper to taste
- Sour cream for serving (optional)
- Fresh dill, chopped, for garnish (optional)

Instructions:

1. In a large pot, heat olive oil over medium heat. Add finely chopped onion, shredded carrots and shredded beets. Cook until the vegetables are softened about 5-7 minutes.
2. Add diced potatoes, shredded cabbage, and minced garlic to the pot. Cook for an additional 5 minutes, stirring frequently.
3. Pour in the vegetable broth and add the diced tomatoes (with their juices) bay leaves, dried dill and apple cider vinegar. Bring the mixture to a simmer.
4. Simmer for about 20-25 minutes or until the vegetables are tender.
5. Season the Vegetarian Borscht with salt and pepper to taste.
6. Remove the bay leaves and discard them.
7. Taste and adjust the seasoning if needed.
8. Ladle the soup into bowls.
9. Optionally, serve with a dollop of sour cream and garnish with chopped fresh dill.
10. Serve the Vegetarian Borscht hot and enjoy the rich and flavorful taste!

Cauliflower and Broccoli Cheese Soup:

Ingredients:

- 2 tablespoons butter

- 1 onion, chopped
- 2 cloves garlic, minced
- 1 head cauliflower, chopped into florets
- 1 head broccoli, chopped into florets
- 4 cups vegetable or chicken broth
- 1 teaspoon dried thyme
- 1 teaspoon dried rosemary
- 1/2 teaspoon smoked paprika
- Salt and pepper to taste
- 2 cups sharp cheddar cheese, shredded
- 1 cup milk (whole or 2%)
- 1/2 cup heavy cream
- Chopped chives for garnish (optional)

Instructions:

1. In a large pot, melt butter over medium heat. Add chopped onion and cook until softened about 5-7 minutes.
2. Add minced garlic and cook for an additional 1-2 minutes, stirring frequently.
3. Add cauliflower and broccoli florets to the pot. Cook for 5 minutes, stirring occasionally.
4. Pour in the vegetable or chicken broth, add dried thyme, dried rosemary, smoked paprika, salt and pepper. Bring the mixture to a simmer.
5. Simmer for about 15-20 minutes or until the cauliflower and broccoli are tender.
6. Use an immersion blender to carefully blend the soup until smooth. Alternatively, transfer the soup in batches to a blender and blend until smooth then return to the pot.
7. Stir in shredded cheddar cheese, milk, and heavy cream. Continue to heat the soup over low heat until the cheese is melted and the soup is heated through.
8. Taste and adjust the seasoning if needed.
9. Ladle the Cauliflower and Broccoli Cheese Soup into bowls.

10. Optionally, garnish with chopped chives.

11. Serve the soup hot and enjoy the creamy and cheesy goodness!

Chicken Tortilla Soup:

Ingredients:

- 1 tablespoon vegetable oil
- 1 onion, diced
- 2 cloves garlic, minced
- 1 teaspoon ground cumin
- 1 teaspoon chili powder
- 1 can (14 oz) diced tomatoes
- 1 can (4 oz) diced green chilies
- 6 cups chicken broth
- 1 pound boneless, skinless chicken breasts, cooked and shredded
- 1 cup corn kernels (fresh or frozen)
- 1 can (15 oz) black beans, drained and rinsed
- 1 teaspoon dried oregano
- Salt and pepper to taste
- Juice of 1 lime
- Tortilla chips, crushed for serving
- Shredded cheese, sour cream, chopped cilantro and sliced green onions for garnish

Instructions:

1. In a large pot, heat vegetable oil over medium heat. Add diced onion and cook until softened about 5 minutes.

2. Add minced garlic, ground cumin, and chili powder to the pot. Cook for an additional 1-2 minutes stirring frequently.

3. Pour in diced tomatoes, diced green chilies and chicken broth. Bring the mixture to a simmer.

4. Add shredded chicken, corn kernels, black beans, dried oregano, salt, and pepper to the pot. Simmer for about 15-20 minutes to allow the flavors to meld.

5. Stir in lime juice and taste the Chicken Tortilla Soup. Adjust the seasoning if needed.

6. Ladle the soup into bowls.

7. Top each serving with crushed tortilla chips, shredded cheese, a dollop of sour cream, chopped cilantro and sliced green onions.

8. Serve the Chicken Tortilla Soup hot and enjoy the delicious combination of flavors and textures!

Sweet Potato and Black Bean Chili:

Ingredients:

- 1 tablespoon olive oil
- 1 onion, diced
- 2 cloves garlic, minced
- 1 large sweet potato, peeled and diced
- 1 red bell pepper, diced
- 1 jalapeño, seeds removed and minced (optional for heat)
- 2 teaspoons ground cumin
- 1 teaspoon chili powder
- 1/2 teaspoon smoked paprika
- 1 can (14 oz) diced tomatoes
- 2 cans (15 oz each) black beans, drained and rinsed
- 3 cups vegetable broth
- Salt and pepper to taste
- Juice of 1 lime
- Fresh cilantro, chopped, for garnish
- Avocado slices for serving (optional)

Instructions:

1. In a large pot, heat olive oil over medium heat. Add diced onion and cook until softened about 5 minutes.

2. Add minced garlic, diced sweet potato, diced red bell pepper, and minced jalapeño (if using) to the pot. Cook for an additional 5 minutes, stirring occasionally.

3. Add ground cumin, chili powder, and smoked paprika to the pot. Stir to coat the vegetables with the spices.

4. Pour in diced tomatoes, black beans, and vegetable broth. Bring the mixture to a simmer.

5. Simmer for about 20-25 minutes or until the sweet potatoes are tender.

6. Season the Sweet Potato and Black Bean Chili with salt, pepper, and lime juice to taste.

7. Taste and adjust the seasoning if needed.

8. Ladle the chili into bowls.

9. Optionally, garnish with chopped fresh cilantro and avocado slices.

10. Serve the Sweet Potato and Black Bean Chili hot and enjoy the hearty and flavorful dish!

Creamy Wild Mushroom Soup:

Ingredients:

- 2 tablespoons butter
- 1 onion, finely chopped
- 2 cloves garlic, minced
- 1 pound (about 454g) mixed wild mushrooms (such as cremini, shiitake, and oyster), cleaned and sliced
- 2 tablespoons all-purpose flour
- 4 cups vegetable or chicken broth
- 1 teaspoon dried thyme
- Salt and pepper to taste
- 1/2 cup heavy cream

- 2 tablespoons dry sherry (optional)
- Chopped fresh parsley for garnish

Instructions:

1. In a large pot, melt butter over medium heat. Add finely chopped onion and cook until softened, about 5-7 minutes.
2. Add minced garlic and sliced wild mushrooms to the pot. Cook for an additional 5 minutes, stirring occasionally.
3. Sprinkle flour over the mushrooms and stir to coat, cooking for 2-3 minutes to remove the raw taste of the flour.
4. Pour in the vegetable or chicken broth, add dried thyme, salt, and pepper. Bring the mixture to a simmer.
5. Simmer for about 15-20 minutes or until the mushrooms are tender.
6. Use an immersion blender to carefully blend the soup until smooth. Alternatively, transfer the soup in batches to a blender and blend until smooth then return to the pot.
7. Stir in heavy cream and dry sherry (if using). Simmer for an additional 5 minutes.
8. Taste and adjust the seasoning if needed.
9. Ladle the Creamy Wild Mushroom Soup into bowls.
10. Optionally, garnish with chopped fresh parsley.
11. Serve the soup hot and enjoy the rich and velvety flavors!

Chickpea and Spinach Stew:

Ingredients:

- 2 tablespoons olive oil
- 1 onion, finely chopped
- 2 cloves garlic, minced
- 1 teaspoon ground cumin
- 1 teaspoon ground coriander
- 1 teaspoon smoked paprika

- 1 can (15 oz) chickpeas, drained and rinsed
- 1 can (14 oz) diced tomatoes
- 4 cups vegetable broth
- 1 bay leaf
- 1 bunch fresh spinach, chopped
- Salt and pepper to taste
- Juice of 1 lemon
- Crumbled feta cheese for serving (optional)

Instructions:

1. In a large pot, heat olive oil over medium heat. Add finely chopped onion and cook until softened about 5-7 minutes.
2. Add minced garlic, ground cumin, ground coriander, and smoked paprika to the pot. Stir and cook for an additional 1-2 minutes.
3. Pour in chickpeas, diced tomatoes (with their juices), vegetable broth and add the bay leaf. Bring the mixture to a simmer.
4. Simmer for about 15-20 minutes to allow the flavors to meld.
5. Stir in chopped fresh spinach and cook until wilted, about 2-3 minutes.
6. Season the Chickpea and Spinach Stew with salt and pepper to taste.
7. Remove the bay leaf and discard it.
8. Stir in lemon juice and taste the stew. Adjust the seasoning if needed.
9. Ladle the stew into bowls.
10. Optionally, top with crumbled feta cheese before serving.
11. Serve the Chickpea and Spinach Stew hot and enjoy this nutritious and flavorful dish!

Stews

Beef and Vegetable Stew:

Ingredients:

- 1.5 pounds (about 680g) beef stew meat, cut into bite-sized pieces
- 2 tablespoons olive oil
- 1 onion, diced
- 2 cloves garlic, minced
- 2 carrots, peeled and sliced
- 2 celery stalks, sliced
- 3 potatoes, peeled and diced
- 1 cup frozen peas
- 1 can (14 oz) diced tomatoes
- 4 cups beef broth
- 1 teaspoon dried thyme
- 1 teaspoon dried rosemary
- Salt and pepper to taste
- 2 tablespoons tomato paste
- 2 tablespoons all-purpose flour
- Chopped fresh parsley for garnish (optional)

Instructions:

1. In a large pot, heat olive oil over medium heat. Add diced onion and cook until softened about 5-7 minutes.
2. Add minced garlic and beef stew meat to the pot. Brown the meat on all sides.
3. Sprinkle flour over the meat and stir to coat, cooking for 2-3 minutes to remove the raw taste of the flour.
4. Pour in beef broth, diced tomatoes (with their juices), dried thyme, dried rosemary, salt and pepper. Bring the mixture to a simmer.
5. Simmer for about 1.5 to 2 hours or until the beef is tender.
6. Add sliced carrots, sliced celery, diced potatoes, frozen peas, and tomato paste to the pot. Simmer for an additional 20-30 minutes or until the vegetables are cooked through.
7. Taste and adjust the seasoning if needed.

8. Ladle the Beef and Vegetable Stew into bowls.

9. Optionally, garnish with chopped fresh parsley.

10. Serve the stew hot and enjoy the hearty and comforting flavors!

Moroccan Chickpea Stew:

Ingredients:

- 2 tablespoons olive oil
- 1 onion, finely chopped
- 2 cloves garlic, minced
- 1 teaspoon ground cumin
- 1 teaspoon ground coriander
- 1 teaspoon smoked paprika
- 1/2 teaspoon ground cinnamon
- 1/2 teaspoon ground turmeric
- 1 can (15 oz) chickpeas, drained and rinsed
- 1 can (14 oz) diced tomatoes
- 4 cups vegetable broth
- 1 sweet potato, peeled and diced
- 1 carrot, peeled and sliced
- 1 zucchini, diced
- 1/2 cup dried apricots, chopped
- Salt and pepper to taste
- 1 cup couscous, cooked (for serving)
- Chopped fresh cilantro for garnish

Instructions:

1. In a large pot, heat olive oil over medium heat. Add finely chopped onion and cook until softened about 5-7 minutes.

2. Add minced garlic, ground cumin, ground coriander, smoked paprika, ground cinnamon, and ground turmeric to the pot. Stir and cook for an additional 1-2 minutes.

3. Pour in chickpeas, diced tomatoes (with their juices), vegetable broth, diced sweet potato, sliced carrot, diced zucchini and chopped dried apricots. Bring the mixture to a simmer.

4. Simmer for about 20-25 minutes or until the vegetables are tender.

5. Season the Moroccan Chickpea Stew with salt and pepper to taste.

6. Taste and adjust the seasoning if needed.

7. While the stew is simmering, cook couscous according to package instructions.

8. Ladle the stew over cooked couscous.

9. Optionally, garnish with chopped fresh cilantro.

10. Serve the Moroccan Chickpea Stew hot and enjoy the aromatic and flavorful dish!

Irish Lamb Stew:

Ingredients:

- 2 pounds (about 907g) lamb stew meat, cut into bite-sized pieces
- 2 tablespoons vegetable oil
- 1 large onion, finely chopped
- 2 cloves garlic, minced
- 4 carrots, peeled and sliced
- 4 potatoes, peeled and diced
- 3 cups beef or lamb broth
- 1 cup Guinness beer (or any stout beer)
- 2 tablespoons tomato paste
- 1 teaspoon dried thyme
- Salt and pepper to taste
- Chopped fresh parsley for garnish

Instructions:

1. In a large pot, heat vegetable oil over medium heat. Add lamb stew meat and brown on all sides.

2. Add finely chopped onion and minced garlic to the pot. Cook until the onion is softened about 5 minutes.

3. Pour in beef or lamb broth, Guinness beer and add tomato paste. Stir to combine.

4. Add sliced carrots, diced potatoes, dried thyme, salt, and pepper to the pot. Bring the mixture to a simmer.

5. Simmer for about 1.5 to 2 hours or until the lamb is tender and the flavors have melded.

6. Taste and adjust the seasoning if needed.

7. Ladle the Irish Lamb Stew into bowls.

8. Optionally, garnish with chopped fresh parsley.

9. Serve the stew hot and enjoy this hearty and traditional Irish dish!

Seafood Cioppino:

Ingredients:

- 2 tablespoons olive oil
- 1 onion, finely chopped
- 2 cloves garlic, minced
- 1/2 teaspoon red pepper flakes (adjust to taste)
- 1 cup white wine
- 1 can (28 oz) crushed tomatoes
- 4 cups fish or seafood broth
- 1 teaspoon dried oregano
- 1 teaspoon dried basil
- Salt and pepper to taste
- 1 pound (about 454g) mixed seafood (such as shrimp, mussels, clams and firm white fish), cleaned and prepared
- 1/2 pound (about 227g) cooked crab meat

- 1/4 cup fresh parsley, chopped
- Crusty bread for serving

Instructions:

1. In a large pot, heat olive oil over medium heat. Add finely chopped onion and cook until softened about 5-7 minutes.
2. Add minced garlic and red pepper flakes to the pot. Cook for an additional 1-2 minutes.
3. Pour in white wine and bring to a simmer. Allow the wine to reduce by half.
4. Add crushed tomatoes, fish or seafood broth, dried oregano, dried basil, salt, and pepper. Bring the mixture to a simmer.
5. Simmer for about 20-25 minutes to allow the flavors to meld.
6. Add mixed seafood and cooked crab meat to the pot. Cook for an additional 5-7 minutes or until the seafood is cooked through.
7. Taste and adjust the seasoning if needed.
8. Stir in chopped fresh parsley.
9. Ladle the Seafood Cioppino into bowls.
10. Serve the Cioppino hot with crusty bread for dipping and enjoy the delicious flavors of the sea!

Vegetable and Lentil Stew:

Ingredients:

- 1 cup dry green or brown lentils, rinsed and drained
- 2 tablespoons olive oil
- 1 onion, finely chopped
- 2 carrots, peeled and diced
- 2 celery stalks, diced
- 3 cloves garlic, minced
- 1 teaspoon ground cumin
- 1 teaspoon ground coriander

- 1 teaspoon smoked paprika
- 1 can (14 oz) diced tomatoes
- 4 cups vegetable broth
- 1 sweet potato, peeled and diced
- 1 zucchini, diced
- 1 cup green beans, trimmed and chopped
- Salt and pepper to taste
- 2 cups spinach or kale, chopped
- Juice of 1 lemon
- Chopped fresh parsley for garnish

Instructions:

1. In a large pot, heat olive oil over medium heat. Add finely chopped onion, diced carrots, and diced celery. Cook until the vegetables are softened about 5-7 minutes.
2. Add minced garlic, ground cumin, ground coriander, and smoked paprika to the pot. Stir and cook for an additional 1-2 minutes.
3. Pour in rinsed lentils, diced tomatoes (with their juices) and vegetable broth. Bring the mixture to a simmer.
4. Simmer for about 15-20 minutes or until the lentils are partially cooked.
5. Add diced sweet potato, diced zucchini and chopped green beans to the pot. Continue to simmer until the lentils and vegetables are tender, about 15-20 minutes more.
6. Season the Vegetable and Lentil Stew with salt and pepper to taste.
7. Stir in chopped spinach or kale and cook until wilted about 2-3 minutes.
8. Remove the pot from heat and stir in lemon juice.
9. Taste and adjust the seasoning if needed.
10. Ladle the stew into bowls.
11. Optionally, garnish with chopped fresh parsley.
12. Serve the Vegetable and Lentil Stew hot and enjoy this nutritious and hearty dish!

Chicken and Dumplings Stew:

Ingredients:

For the Stew:

- 2 tablespoons butter
- 1 onion, finely chopped
- 2 carrots, peeled and sliced
- 2 celery stalks, sliced
- 3 cloves garlic, minced
- 1 teaspoon dried thyme
- 1 teaspoon dried rosemary
- 1/2 cup all-purpose flour
- 4 cups chicken broth
- 1.5 pounds boneless, skinless chicken thighs cut into bite-sized pieces
- Salt and pepper to taste
- 1 cup frozen peas
- 1 cup frozen corn
- 1/2 cup heavy cream

For the Dumplings:

- 2 cups all-purpose flour
- 1 tablespoon baking powder
- 1/2 teaspoon salt
- 1 cup milk
- 1/4 cup fresh parsley, chopped

Instructions:

For the Stew:

1. In a large pot, melt butter over medium heat. Add finely chopped onion, sliced carrots, sliced celery and minced garlic. Cook until the vegetables are softened about 5-7 minutes.

2. Add dried thyme, dried rosemary and flour to the pot. Stir to coat the vegetables with the flour.

3. Pour in chicken broth and stir until the mixture thickens.

4. Add chicken pieces to the pot. Season with salt and pepper to taste.

5. Simmer for about 20-25 minutes or until the chicken is cooked through.

6. Stir in frozen peas, frozen corn and heavy cream. Simmer for an additional 5-7 minutes.

For the Dumplings:

1. In a bowl, whisk together flour, baking powder, and salt.

2. Add milk and chopped parsley to the dry ingredients. Stir until just combined.

3. Drop spoonfuls of the dumpling batter onto the simmering stew.

4. Cover the pot and let the dumplings cook for 15-20 minutes or until they are cooked through and fluffy.

5. Serve the Chicken and Dumplings Stew hot with a spoonful of dumplings in each bowl.

Brazilian Feijoada:

Ingredients:

- 1 pound (about 454g) black beans, dried
- 2 tablespoons vegetable oil
- 1 onion, finely chopped
- 4 cloves garlic, minced
- 1 pound (about 454g) pork shoulder, cut into chunks
- 1/2 pound (about 227g) smoked sausage, sliced
- 1/2 pound (about 227g) chorizo sausage, sliced
- 1/2 pound (about 227g) bacon, chopped
- 2 bay leaves
- 1 teaspoon cumin
- 1 teaspoon paprika

- Salt and pepper to taste
- 4 cups water
- Rice for serving
- Fresh orange slices for garnish

Instructions:

1. Rinse the black beans under cold water and soak them overnight. Alternatively, you can use the quick soak method by boiling the beans for 2 minutes and then letting them soak for 1 hour.
2. In a large pot, heat vegetable oil over medium heat. Add finely chopped onion and minced garlic. Cook until the onion is softened about 5 minutes.
3. Add pork shoulder chunks, sliced smoked sausage, sliced chorizo sausage and chopped bacon to the pot. Brown the meat for about 5-7 minutes.
4. Stir in soaked black beans, bay leaves, cumin, paprika, salt and pepper. Mix well to combine.
5. Pour in water and bring the mixture to a boil.
6. Reduce the heat to low, cover the pot and simmer for about 2-3 hours or until the beans are tender and the meat is cooked through.
7. Adjust the seasoning if needed.
8. Serve the Brazilian Feijoada over rice and garnish with fresh orange slices.
9. Enjoy this hearty and flavorful Brazilian dish!

Spicy Pumpkin and Black Bean Stew:

Ingredients:

- 2 tablespoons olive oil
- 1 onion, finely chopped
- 2 cloves garlic, minced
- 1 jalapeño, seeds removed and minced
- 1 teaspoon ground cumin
- 1 teaspoon chili powder

- 1/2 teaspoon smoked paprika
- 1/4 teaspoon cayenne pepper (adjust to taste)
- 1 can (15 oz) black beans, drained and rinsed
- 1 can (15 oz) diced tomatoes
- 1 can (15 oz) pumpkin puree
- 4 cups vegetable broth
- 1 cup corn kernels (fresh or frozen)
- Salt and pepper to taste
- Juice of 1 lime
- Chopped fresh cilantro for garnish
- Sour cream or Greek yogurt for serving (optional)

Instructions:

1. In a large pot, heat olive oil over medium heat. Add finely chopped onion and cook until softened, about 5-7 minutes.
2. Add minced garlic and minced jalapeño to the pot. Cook for an additional 1-2 minutes.
3. Stir in ground cumin, chili powder, smoked paprika and cayenne pepper to the pot. Mix well to coat the vegetables with the spices.
4. Add black beans, diced tomatoes (with their juices), pumpkin puree and vegetable broth. Bring the mixture to a simmer.
5. Simmer for about 15-20 minutes to allow the flavors to meld.
6. Add corn kernels to the pot and cook for an additional 5 minutes.
7. Season the Spicy Pumpkin and Black Bean Stew with salt, pepper and lime juice to taste.
8. Taste and adjust the seasoning if needed.
9. Ladle the stew into bowls.
10. Optionally, garnish with chopped fresh cilantro and a dollop of sour cream or Greek yogurt.

11. Serve the Spicy Pumpkin and Black Bean Stew hot and enjoy the bold and warming flavors!

Venison and Root Vegetable Stew:

Ingredients:

- 2 pounds (about 907g) venison stew meat cut into bite-sized pieces
- 2 tablespoons vegetable oil
- 1 onion, finely chopped
- 3 cloves garlic, minced
- 4 carrots, peeled and sliced
- 3 parsnips, peeled and sliced
- 2 turnips, peeled and diced
- 4 cups beef or venison broth
- 1 cup red wine (optional)
- 2 bay leaves
- 1 teaspoon dried thyme
- Salt and pepper to taste
- 2 tablespoons tomato paste
- 1 tablespoon Worcestershire sauce
- 1 cup frozen peas
- Chopped fresh parsley for garnish

Instructions:

1. In a large pot, heat vegetable oil over medium heat. Add finely chopped onion and cook until softened, about 5-7 minutes.
2. Add minced garlic and venison stew meat to the pot. Brown the meat on all sides.
3. Pour in beef or venison broth, red wine (if using), bay leaves, dried thyme, salt and pepper. Bring the mixture to a simmer.
4. Simmer for about 1.5 to 2 hours or until the venison is tender.

5. Add sliced carrots, sliced parsnips, diced turnips, tomato paste and Worcestershire sauce to the pot. Simmer for an additional 30-40 minutes or until the vegetables are cooked through.

6. Stir in frozen peas and cook for an additional 5 minutes.

7. Taste and adjust the seasoning if needed.

8. Remove the bay leaves and discard them.

9. Ladle the Venison and Root Vegetable Stew into bowls.

10. Optionally, garnish with chopped fresh parsley.

11. Serve the stew hot and enjoy the rich and hearty flavors!

Italian Wedding Soup:

Ingredients:

For the Meatballs:

- 1/2 pound (about 227g) ground beef
- 1/2 pound (about 227g) ground pork
- 1/2 cup breadcrumbs
- 1/4 cup grated Parmesan cheese
- 1/4 cup fresh parsley, chopped
- 1 clove garlic, minced
- 1 egg
- Salt and pepper to taste

For the Soup:

- 2 tablespoons olive oil
- 1 onion, finely chopped
- 2 carrots, peeled and sliced
- 2 celery stalks, sliced
- 3 cloves garlic, minced
- 8 cups chicken broth
- 1 teaspoon dried oregano

- 1 teaspoon dried thyme
- Salt and pepper to taste
- 1 cup acini di pepe pasta (or small pasta of your choice)
- 4 cups fresh spinach or kale, chopped
- Grated Parmesan cheese for serving

Instructions:

For the Meatballs:

1. Preheat the oven to 375°F (190°C).
2. In a bowl, combine ground beef, ground pork, breadcrumbs, grated Parmesan cheese, chopped fresh parsley, minced garlic, egg, salt and pepper. Mix until well combined.
3. Shape the mixture into small meatballs about 1 inch in diameter.
4. Place the meatballs on a baking sheet and bake in the preheated oven for 15-20 minutes or until cooked through and browned.

For the Soup:

1. In a large pot, heat olive oil over medium heat. Add finely chopped onion, sliced carrots, sliced celery, and minced garlic. Cook until the vegetables are softened about 5-7 minutes.
2. Pour in chicken broth and add dried oregano, dried thyme, salt and pepper. Bring the mixture to a simmer.
3. Add acini di pepe pasta (or your chosen small pasta) to the pot. Cook according to the package instructions.
4. Once the pasta is almost done, stir in the chopped fresh spinach or kale and the baked meatballs. Simmer for an additional 5-7 minutes.
5. Taste and adjust the seasoning if needed.
6. Ladle the Italian Wedding Soup into bowls.
7. Optionally, sprinkle each serving with grated Parmesan cheese.
8. Serve the soup hot and enjoy the comforting and flavorful dish!

Asian-Inspired Tofu and Vegetable Stew:

Ingredients:

- 1 block (about 14 oz) firm tofu, pressed and cubed
- 2 tablespoons soy sauce
- 1 tablespoon sesame oil
- 2 tablespoons vegetable oil
- 1 onion, thinly sliced
- 2 carrots, julienned
- 1 red bell pepper, thinly sliced
- 1 zucchini, thinly sliced
- 3 cloves garlic, minced
- 1 tablespoon fresh ginger, grated
- 4 cups vegetable broth
- 2 tablespoons miso paste
- 1 tablespoon rice vinegar
- 1 tablespoon soy sauce (additional)
- 1 teaspoon Sriracha sauce (adjust to taste)
- 1 cup shiitake mushrooms, sliced
- 1 cup baby spinach
- Green onions, sliced for garnish
- Cooked rice or rice noodles for serving

Instructions:

1. In a bowl, toss the cubed tofu with soy sauce and sesame oil. Allow it to marinate while you prepare the vegetables.
2. In a large pot, heat vegetable oil over medium heat. Add thinly sliced onion, julienned carrots, sliced red bell pepper and sliced zucchini. Saute until the vegetables are softened about 5-7 minutes.
3. Add minced garlic and grated ginger to the pot. Cook for an additional 1-2 minutes until fragrant.

4. Pour in vegetable broth, miso paste, rice vinegar additional soy sauce and Sriracha sauce. Stir to combine.

5. Add the marinated tofu and sliced shiitake mushrooms to the pot. Simmer for about 10-15 minutes to allow the flavors to meld.

6. Taste the stew and adjust the seasoning if needed.

7. Just before serving, stir in baby spinach until wilted.

8. Serve the Asian-Inspired Tofu and Vegetable Stew over cooked rice or rice noodles.

9. Garnish with sliced green onions.

10. Enjoy this flavorful and nourishing stew!

Spanish Seafood Stew (Zarzuela):

Ingredients:

- 2 tablespoons olive oil
- 1 onion, finely chopped
- 3 cloves garlic, minced
- 1 red bell pepper, thinly sliced
- 1 green bell pepper, thinly sliced
- 1 fennel bulb, thinly sliced
- 1 teaspoon smoked paprika
- 1/2 teaspoon saffron threads
- 1 cup dry white wine
- 1 can (14 oz) diced tomatoes
- 4 cups fish or seafood broth
- 1 bay leaf
- Salt and pepper to taste
- 1 pound mixed seafood (such as shrimp, mussels, clams and firm white fish), cleaned and prepared
- 1/2 cup fresh parsley, chopped

- Crusty bread for serving

Instructions:

1. In a large pot, heat olive oil over medium heat. Add finely chopped onion and cook until softened about 5-7 minutes.
2. Add minced garlic, thinly sliced red and green bell peppers and thinly sliced fennel to the pot. Cook until the vegetables are softened about 5 minutes.
3. Stir in smoked paprika and saffron threads to the pot. Mix well to coat the vegetables with the spices.
4. Pour in dry white wine and bring the mixture to a simmer. Allow the wine to reduce by half.
5. Add diced tomatoes (with their juices), fish or seafood broth, bay leaf, salt and pepper to the pot. Bring the mixture to a simmer.
6. Simmer for about 20-25 minutes to allow the flavors to meld.
7. Add mixed seafood to the pot. Cook for an additional 5-7 minutes or until the seafood is cooked through. Discard any unopened mussels or clams.
8. Taste and adjust the seasoning if needed.
9. Stir in chopped fresh parsley.
10. Ladle the Spanish Seafood Stew (Zarzuela) into bowls.
11. Serve the stew hot with crusty bread for dipping, and enjoy the rich and vibrant flavors!

Barbecue Chicken and Black-Eyed Pea Stew:

Ingredients:

- 1.5 pounds boneless, skinless chicken thighs cut into bite-sized pieces
- 2 tablespoons vegetable oil
- 1 onion, finely chopped
- 2 cloves garlic, minced
- 1 red bell pepper, diced
- 1 can (15 oz) black-eyed peas, drained and rinsed

- 1 can (14 oz) diced tomatoes
- 1/2 cup barbecue sauce
- 4 cups chicken broth
- 1 teaspoon smoked paprika
- 1 teaspoon chili powder
- Salt and pepper to taste
- 1 cup corn kernels (fresh or frozen)
- Chopped fresh cilantro for garnish
- Cooked rice for serving

Instructions:

1. In a large pot, heat vegetable oil over medium heat. Add finely chopped onion, minced garlic and diced red bell pepper. Cook until the vegetables are softened, about 5-7 minutes.
2. Add bite-sized chicken pieces to the pot. Brown the chicken on all sides.
3. Stir in black-eyed peas, diced tomatoes (with their juices), barbecue sauce, chicken broth, smoked paprika, chili powder, salt and pepper. Bring the mixture to a simmer.
4. Simmer for about 20-25 minutes to allow the flavors to meld.
5. Add corn kernels to the pot and cook for an additional 5 minutes.
6. Taste and adjust the seasoning if needed.
7. Ladle the Barbecue Chicken and Black-Eyed Pea Stew into bowls.
8. Optionally, garnish with chopped fresh cilantro.
9. Serve the stew hot over cooked rice and enjoy the delicious barbecue-infused flavors!

Sweet and Sour Cabbage Roll Stew:

Ingredients:

- 1 pound ground beef or ground turkey
- 1 onion, finely chopped

- 2 cloves garlic, minced
- 1 cup cooked rice
- 1 head cabbage, shredded
- 1 can (14 oz) diced tomatoes
- 1 can (8 oz) tomato sauce
- 1/2 cup apple cider vinegar
- 1/4 cup brown sugar
- 2 tablespoons soy sauce
- 1 teaspoon paprika
- Salt and pepper to taste
- 4 cups beef or vegetable broth
- Chopped fresh parsley for garnish

Instructions:

1. In a large pot, cook ground beef or turkey over medium heat until browned. Drain any excess fat.
2. Add finely chopped onion and minced garlic to the pot. Cook until the onion is softened about 5-7 minutes.
3. Stir in cooked rice, shredded cabbage, diced tomatoes (with their juices) tomato sauce, apple cider vinegar, brown sugar, soy sauce, paprika, salt and pepper. Mix well to combine.
4. Pour in beef or vegetable broth. Bring the mixture to a simmer.
5. Simmer for about 25-30 minutes or until the cabbage is tender.
6. Taste and adjust the seasoning if needed.
7. Ladle the Sweet and Sour Cabbage Roll Stew into bowls.
8. Optionally, garnish with chopped fresh parsley.
9. Serve the stew hot and enjoy the sweet and tangy flavors reminiscent of cabbage rolls!

Chicken, Quinoa and Vegetable Stew:

Ingredients:

- 1 pound boneless, skinless chicken thighs cut into bite-sized pieces
- 2 tablespoons olive oil
- 1 onion, finely chopped
- 2 carrots, peeled and diced
- 2 celery stalks, diced
- 3 cloves garlic, minced
- 1 teaspoon dried thyme
- 1 teaspoon dried rosemary
- 1 cup quinoa, rinsed
- 4 cups chicken broth
- 1 can (14 oz) diced tomatoes
- 1 zucchini, diced
- 1 cup green beans, trimmed and chopped
- Salt and pepper to taste
- 2 cups spinach or kale chopped
- Juice of 1 lemon
- Chopped fresh parsley for garnish

Instructions:

1. In a large pot, heat olive oil over medium heat. Add finely chopped onion, diced carrots and diced celery. Cook until the vegetables are softened about 5-7 minutes.
2. Add minced garlic, dried thyme, and dried rosemary to the pot. Stir and cook for an additional 1-2 minutes until fragrant.
3. Add chicken pieces to the pot. Brown the chicken on all sides.
4. Stir in quinoa, chicken broth, diced tomatoes (with their juices), diced zucchini and chopped green beans. Bring the mixture to a simmer.
5. Simmer for about 15-20 minutes or until the quinoa is cooked and the chicken is tender.

6. Season the Chicken, Quinoa and Vegetable Stew with salt and pepper to taste.

7. Stir in chopped spinach or kale and cook until wilted, about 2-3 minutes.

8. Remove the pot from heat and stir in lemon juice.

9. Taste and adjust the seasoning if needed.

10. Ladle the stew into bowls.

11. Optionally, garnish with chopped fresh parsley.

12. Serve the Chicken Quinoa, and Vegetable Stew hot and enjoy this wholesome and nutritious dish!

CHAPTER 9: WEEKLY MEAL PLANS

Day 1:

Breakfast: Green smoothie with spinach, cucumber, celery, green apple and a teaspoon of chia seeds.

Ingredients:

- 1 cup fresh spinach leaves, washed
- 1/2 cucumber, peeled and sliced
- 2 celery stalks, chopped
- 1 green apple, cored and chopped
- 1 teaspoon chia seeds
- 1 cup cold water or coconut water
- Ice cubes (optional)

Instructions:

1. Place fresh spinach leaves, sliced cucumber, chopped celery, chopped green apple and chia seeds in a blender.
2. Add cold water or coconut water to the blender.
3. Blend the ingredients on high speed until the mixture is smooth and well combined.
4. If you prefer a colder smoothie, you can add ice cubes to the blender and blend again until the desired consistency is reached.
5. Pour the green smoothie into a glass.
6. Optionally, sprinkle additional chia seeds on top for texture.
7. Stir before drinking as chia seeds may settle at the bottom.
8. Enjoy your refreshing and nutritious green smoothie!

Lunch: Quinoa salad with mixed vegetables (carrots, bell peppers, cherry tomatoes) and a light olive oil dressing.

Ingredients:

For the Quinoa Salad:

- 1 cup quinoa, rinsed
- 2 cups water
- 1 cup cherry tomatoes, halved
- 1 cup carrots, diced
- 1 cup bell peppers (mixed colors), diced
- Fresh parsley or cilantro, chopped (for garnish)

For the Olive Oil Dressing:

- 3 tablespoons extra virgin olive oil
- 1 tablespoon balsamic vinegar
- 1 teaspoon Dijon mustard
- 1 clove garlic, minced
- Salt and pepper to taste

Instructions:

1. In a medium saucepan, combine quinoa and water. Bring to a boil, then reduce the heat to low, cover and simmer for 15 minutes or until the quinoa is cooked and water is absorbed. Remove from heat and let it cool.

2. In a large bowl, combine the cooked and cooled quinoa with cherry tomatoes, diced carrots and diced bell peppers.

3. In a small bowl or jar whisk together extra virgin olive oil, balsamic vinegar, Dijon mustard, minced garlic, salt and pepper to create the dressing.

4. Pour the olive oil dressing over the quinoa and vegetable mixture. Toss gently to coat everything evenly.

5. Let the quinoa salad sit for a few minutes to allow the flavors to meld.

6. Garnish with fresh parsley or cilantro.

7. Taste and adjust the seasoning if needed.

8. Serve the Quinoa Salad with Mixed Vegetables at room temperature or chilled.

9. Enjoy this light and nutritious salad as a side dish or a main meal!

Dinner: Grilled chicken or tofu with steamed broccoli and a side of brown rice.

Ingredients:

For Grilled Chicken or Tofu:

- 1 pound boneless, skinless chicken breasts or extra-firm tofu
- 2 tablespoons olive oil
- 1 teaspoon garlic powder
- 1 teaspoon paprika
- Salt and pepper to taste

For Steamed Broccoli:

- 2 cups broccoli florets
- 1 tablespoon olive oil
- Salt and pepper to taste

For Brown Rice:

- 1 cup brown rice
- 2 cups water
- 1/2 teaspoon salt

Instructions:

Grilled Chicken or Tofu:

1. If using chicken, preheat the grill to medium-high heat. If using tofu, preheat a grill pan or skillet.

2. In a bowl, mix olive oil, garlic powder, paprika, salt and pepper to create a marinade.

3. Coat the chicken breasts or tofu with the marinade, ensuring even coverage.

4. Grill the chicken for about 6-8 minutes per side or until cooked through. For tofu grill for 4-5 minutes per side until grill marks appear.

5. Once cooked, let the chicken or tofu rest for a few minutes before slicing.

Steamed Broccoli:

1. In a steamer basket over boiling water, steam broccoli florets for 3-5 minutes or until crisp-tender.
2. Drizzle olive oil over the steamed broccoli and season with salt and pepper.

Brown Rice:

1. Rinse the brown rice under cold water.
2. In a saucepan, bring 2 cups of water to a boil. Add the rinsed brown rice and salt.
3. Reduce heat to low, cover and simmer for about 45-50 minutes or until the rice is tender and water is absorbed.

Assembling the Dish:

1. Serve the grilled chicken or tofu slices on a plate.
2. Arrange the steamed broccoli on the side.
3. Serve a portion of brown rice alongside the chicken or tofu.
4. Optionally, drizzle a bit of olive oil over the rice and sprinkle with additional salt and pepper for added flavor.
5. Enjoy your wholesome and balanced meal!

Day 2:

Breakfast: Fresh fruit salad with berries, melon and citrus fruits.

Ingredients:

- 1 cup strawberries, hulled and halved
- 1 cup blueberries
- 1 cup raspberries
- 1 cup blackberries
- 2 cups cubed watermelon
- 2 cups cubed cantaloupe or honeydew melon
- 2 oranges, peeled and segmented

- 1 grapefruit, peeled and segmented
- Fresh mint leaves for garnish (optional)

For Citrus Honey Dressing:

- 2 tablespoons honey
- 2 tablespoons fresh orange juice
- 1 tablespoon fresh lemon juice
- Zest of 1 orange
- Zest of 1 lemon

Instructions:

1. In a large bowl, combine strawberries, blueberries, raspberries, blackberries, watermelon cubes, cantaloupe or honeydew cubes, orange segments and grapefruit segments.
2. In a separate small bowl, whisk together honey, fresh orange juice, fresh lemon juice, orange zest and lemon zest to create the citrus honey dressing.
3. Drizzle the citrus honey dressing over the fresh fruit in the large bowl.
4. Gently toss the fruit salad until well coated with the dressing.
5. Let the fruit salad sit for a few minutes to allow the flavors to meld.
6. Optionally, garnish with fresh mint leaves for added freshness.
7. Serve the Fresh Fruit Salad immediately and enjoy the vibrant and refreshing combination of berries, melon and citrus fruits!

Lunch: Lentil soup with plenty of leafy greens like kale or spinach.

Ingredients:

- 1 cup dried green or brown lentils, rinsed and drained
- 1 onion, finely chopped
- 2 carrots, diced
- 2 celery stalks, diced
- 3 cloves garlic, minced
- 1 teaspoon ground cumin

- 1 teaspoon ground coriander
- 1 teaspoon smoked paprika
- 6 cups vegetable broth
- 1 can (14 oz) diced tomatoes
- 2 cups chopped kale or spinach
- Salt and pepper to taste
- 2 tablespoons olive oil
- Lemon wedges for serving (optional)

Instructions:

1. In a large pot, heat olive oil over medium heat. Add finely chopped onion, diced carrots and diced celery. Cook until the vegetables are softened about 5-7 minutes.
2. Add minced garlic, ground cumin, ground coriander, and smoked paprika to the pot. Stir and cook for an additional 1-2 minutes until fragrant.
3. Pour in vegetable broth and add rinsed lentils. Bring the mixture to a boil.
4. Reduce the heat to low, cover the pot and simmer for about 20-25 minutes or until the lentils are tender.
5. Add diced tomatoes (with their juices) to the pot. Stir to combine.
6. Stir in chopped kale or spinach. Simmer for an additional 5-7 minutes until the greens are wilted.
7. Season the lentil soup with salt and pepper to taste.
8. Taste and adjust the seasoning if needed.
9. Ladle the Lentil Soup with Leafy Greens into bowls.
10. Optionally, squeeze a bit of lemon juice over each serving for added freshness.
11. Serve the soup hot and enjoy this hearty and nutritious dish!

Dinner: Baked salmon with roasted sweet potatoes and asparagus.

Ingredients:

For Baked Salmon:

- 4 salmon filets (about 6 oz each)

- 2 tablespoons olive oil

- 2 cloves garlic, minced

- 1 teaspoon dried oregano

- 1 teaspoon dried thyme

- 1 teaspoon paprika

- Salt and pepper to taste

- Lemon wedges for serving (optional)

For Roasted Sweet Potatoes and Asparagus:

- 2 large sweet potatoes, peeled and diced

- 1 bunch asparagus, trimmed

- 2 tablespoons olive oil

- Salt and pepper to taste

- 1 teaspoon garlic powder

- 1 teaspoon dried rosemary

Instructions:

Baked Salmon:

1. Preheat the oven to 400°F (200°C).

2. Place salmon filets on a baking sheet lined with parchment paper.

3. In a small bowl, mix olive oil, minced garlic, dried oregano, dried thyme, paprika, salt and pepper to create a marinade.

4. Brush the salmon filets with the marinade ensuring they are well-coated.

5. Bake the salmon in the preheated oven for about 12-15 minutes or until the salmon easily flakes with a fork.

6. Optionally, squeeze lemon wedges over the baked salmon before serving.

Roasted Sweet Potatoes and Asparagus:

1. In a large bowl, toss diced sweet potatoes and trimmed asparagus with olive oil.

2. Season with salt, pepper, garlic powder and dried rosemary. Toss to coat evenly.

3. Spread the sweet potatoes and asparagus on a separate baking sheet lined with parchment paper.

4. Roast in the preheated oven for about 20-25 minutes or until the sweet potatoes are tender and the asparagus is slightly crispy.

Assembling the Dish:

1. Serve the baked salmon filets on plates.
2. Arrange the roasted sweet potatoes and asparagus alongside the salmon.
3. Optionally, garnish with additional herbs or a squeeze of lemon.
4. Enjoy your flavorful and nutritious Baked Salmon with Roasted Sweet Potatoes and Asparagus!

Day 3:

Breakfast: Overnight oats made with almond milk, topped with sliced bananas and a sprinkle of pumpkin seeds.

Ingredients:

- 1/2 cup rolled oats
- 1/2 cup almond milk (or any milk of your choice)
- 1 tablespoon chia seeds
- 1/2 teaspoon vanilla extract
- 1-2 tablespoons maple syrup or honey (optional, for sweetness)
- 1 ripe banana, sliced
- 1 tablespoon pumpkin seeds (pepitas)

Instructions:

1. In a jar or airtight container, combine rolled oats, almond milk, chia seeds, vanilla extract and maple syrup (if using).
2. Stir the mixture well to ensure the oats and chia seeds are evenly distributed and submerged in the liquid.
3. Seal the jar or container and refrigerate overnight or for at least 4 hours. This allows the oats and chia seeds to absorb the liquid and create a creamy texture.

4. In the morning or when ready to eat, give the overnight oats a good stir. If the mixture is too thick, you can add a splash of additional almond milk to reach your desired consistency.

5. Top the overnight oats with sliced bananas and sprinkle pumpkin seeds on top.

6. Optionally, drizzle with a bit more maple syrup or honey for added sweetness.

7. Enjoy your delicious and convenient Overnight Oats with Almond Milk, Sliced Bananas and Pumpkin Seeds!

Lunch: Chickpea salad with diced cucumbers, cherry tomatoes, red onion and a lemon-tahini dressing.

Ingredients:

For Chickpea Salad:

- 2 cans (15 oz each) chickpeas, drained and rinsed
- 1 cucumber, diced
- 1 cup cherry tomatoes, halved
- 1/2 red onion, finely chopped
- 1/4 cup fresh parsley, chopped

For Lemon-Tahini Dressing:

- 3 tablespoons tahini
- Juice of 1 lemon
- 2 tablespoons olive oil
- 1 clove garlic, minced
- Salt and pepper to taste
- Water (to thin the dressing, if needed)

Instructions:

Chickpea Salad:

1. In a large bowl, combine chickpeas, diced cucumber, cherry tomatoes, chopped red onion and fresh parsley.

2. Toss the ingredients together until well mixed.

Lemon-Tahini Dressing:

1. In a small bowl, whisk together tahini, lemon juice, olive oil, minced garlic, salt, and pepper.
2. If the dressing is too thick, you can add a little water to reach your desired consistency. Start with a tablespoon and add more as needed.
3. Taste the dressing and adjust the seasoning if needed.

Assembling the Chickpea Salad:

1. Pour the Lemon-Tahini Dressing over the chickpea salad.
2. Toss the salad until the ingredients are evenly coated with the dressing.
3. Let the chickpea salad sit for a few minutes to allow the flavors to meld.
4. Optionally, garnish with additional fresh parsley.
5. Serve the Chickpea Salad with Lemon-Tahini Dressing as a side dish or a light and satisfying main meal.

Dinner: Stir-fried tofu with broccoli, bok choy and shiitake mushrooms served over quinoa.

Ingredients:

For Stir-Fried Tofu:

- 1 block extra-firm tofu, pressed and cubed
- 2 tablespoons soy sauce
- 1 tablespoon sesame oil
- 1 tablespoon cornstarch
- 1 tablespoon vegetable oil (for cooking)

For Stir-Fry Vegetables:

- 1 cup broccoli florets
- 2 baby bok choy, chopped
- 1 cup shiitake mushrooms, sliced
- 2 cloves garlic, minced
- 1 tablespoon ginger, grated

- 2 tablespoons soy sauce
- 1 tablespoon hoisin sauce
- 1 tablespoon rice vinegar
- 1 tablespoon sesame oil

For Serving:

- 2 cups cooked quinoa

Instructions:

Stir-Fried Tofu:

1. In a bowl, combine cubed tofu with soy sauce, sesame oil, and cornstarch. Toss gently to coat the tofu evenly.
2. Heat vegetable oil in a wok or large skillet over medium-high heat.
3. Add the tofu to the hot pan and stir-fry until golden brown on all sides. This usually takes about 8-10 minutes. Set aside.

Stir-Fry Vegetables:

1. In the same wok or skillet, add a bit more vegetable oil if needed.
2. Add minced garlic and grated ginger, stir-frying for about 30 seconds until fragrant.
3. Add broccoli florets, chopped bok choy and sliced shiitake mushrooms to the pan. Stir-fry for another 3-5 minutes until the vegetables are slightly tender but still crisp.
4. Combine soy sauce, hoisin sauce, rice vinegar, and sesame oil in a small bowl. Pour the sauce over the vegetables in the wok.
5. Add the stir-fried tofu back into the wok and toss everything together until well coated with the sauce. Cook for an additional 2-3 minutes to heat through.

Serving:

1. Serve the stir-fried tofu, broccoli, bok choy and shiitake mushrooms over cooked quinoa.
2. Optionally, garnish with sesame seeds or chopped green onions.

3. Enjoy this flavorful and protein-packed Stir-Fried Tofu with Quinoa and Mixed Vegetables!

Breakfast: Whole grain toast with avocado and cherry tomatoes.

Ingredients:

- 2 slices whole grain bread, toasted
- 1 ripe avocado
- 1 cup cherry tomatoes, halved
- Salt and pepper to taste
- Red pepper flakes (optional, for added heat)
- Fresh cilantro or basil leaves for garnish (optional)
- Drizzle of olive oil (optional)

Instructions:

1. Toast the whole grain bread slices to your desired level of crispiness.
2. While the bread is toasting, cut the avocado in half, remove the pit and scoop the flesh into a bowl.
3. Mash the avocado with a fork until you achieve your preferred level of creaminess. You can leave it slightly chunky or make it smoother.
4. Spread the mashed avocado evenly over the toasted whole grain bread slices.
5. Top the avocado-covered toast with halved cherry tomatoes, distributing them evenly.
6. Season the toast with salt and pepper to taste. If you enjoy some heat, sprinkle red pepper flakes over the top.
7. Optionally, garnish with fresh cilantro or basil leaves for added flavor.
8. For an extra touch, drizzle a bit of olive oil over the avocado and tomatoes.
9. Serve the Whole Grain Toast with Avocado and Cherry Tomatoes immediately.
10. Enjoy this simple and nutritious toast as a quick breakfast.

Lunch: Brown rice bowl with black beans, corn, diced avocado and a squeeze of lime.

Ingredients:

- 1 cup cooked brown rice
- 1 can (15 oz) black beans, drained and rinsed
- 1 cup corn kernels (fresh, frozen, or canned)
- 1 ripe avocado, diced
- 1 lime, cut into wedges
- Fresh cilantro, chopped (optional, for garnish)
- Salt and pepper to taste

Instructions:

1. In a bowl, layer cooked brown rice as the base.
2. Add black beans on top of the brown rice.
3. Add corn kernels on the other side of the bowl.
4. Dice the ripe avocado and place it in the bowl.
5. Squeeze lime wedges over the entire rice bowl for a citrusy flavor.
6. Season the bowl with salt and pepper to taste.
7. Optionally, garnish with chopped fresh cilantro for added freshness.
8. Toss the ingredients gently to combine or keep them separate for a visually appealing bowl.
9. Serve the Brown Rice Bowl with Black Beans, Corn, Diced Avocado and a Squeeze of Lime.

Dinner: Grilled chicken or tempeh with a mixed green salad and a simple vinaigrette dressing.

Ingredients:

For Grilled Chicken or Tempeh:

- 4 boneless, skinless chicken breasts OR 1 package tempeh, sliced
- 2 tablespoons olive oil

* 1 teaspoon dried oregano

* 1 teaspoon smoked paprika

* Salt and pepper to taste

For Mixed Green Salad:

* 6 cups mixed salad greens (lettuce, spinach, arugula, etc.)

* 1 cup cherry tomatoes, halved

* 1 cucumber, sliced

* 1/2 red onion, thinly sliced

* 1 cup sliced bell peppers (mixed colors)

* 1/4 cup sliced black olives (optional)

For Vinaigrette Dressing:

* 3 tablespoons balsamic vinegar

* 1/4 cup extra virgin olive oil

* 1 teaspoon Dijon mustard

* 1 clove garlic, minced

* Salt and pepper to taste

Instructions:

Grilled Chicken or Tempeh:

1. If using chicken, preheat the grill to medium-high heat. If using tempeh preheat a grill pan or skillet.

2. In a bowl, mix olive oil, dried oregano, smoked paprika, salt and pepper to create a marinade.

3. Coat the chicken breasts or tempeh slices with the marinadeensuring even coverage.

4. Grill the chicken for about 6-8 minutes per side or until cooked through. For tempeh, grill for 3-4 minutes per side until grill marks appear.

5. Once cooked, let the chicken or tempeh rest for a few minutes before slicing.

Mixed Green Salad:

1. In a large salad bowl, combine mixed salad greens, cherry tomatoes, sliced cucumber, thinly sliced red onion, sliced bell peppers and black olives (if using).

Vinaigrette Dressing:

1. In a small bowl or jar whisk together balsamic vinegar, extra virgin olive oil, Dijon mustard, minced garlic, salt and pepper.
2. Taste the dressing and adjust the seasoning if needed.

Assembling the Dish:

1. Arrange the grilled chicken or tempeh slices on top of the mixed green salad.
2. Drizzle the vinaigrette dressing over the salad and protein.
3. Toss the salad gently to coat everything with the dressing.
4. Optionally, garnish with additional herbs or a sprinkle of feta cheese.
5. Serve the Grilled Chicken or Tempeh with Mixed Green Salad and Vinaigrette Dressing.

Day 5:

Breakfast: Greek yogurt parfait with fresh berries, a drizzle of honey and a handful of almonds.

Ingredients:

- 1 cup Greek yogurt
- 1 cup mixed fresh berries (strawberries, blueberries, raspberries, blackberries)
- 2 tablespoons honey
- 1/4 cup almonds, sliced or chopped

Instructions:

1. In a glass or a bowl, start by layering about 1/4 cup of Greek yogurt at the bottom.
2. Add a layer of mixed fresh berries on top of the yogurt.
3. Drizzle a tablespoon of honey over the berries.
4. Sprinkle a handful of sliced or chopped almonds over the honey.
5. Repeat the layers until you reach the top of the glass or bowl.

6. Finish with a final drizzle of honey and a few additional berries and almonds for garnish.

7. Serve the Greek Yogurt Parfait immediately and enjoy the delightful combination of creamy yogurt, sweet berries, crunchy almonds and the natural sweetness of honey!

Lunch: Spinach and kale salad with grilled shrimp, cherry tomatoes and a light olive oil dressing.

Ingredients:

For Grilled Shrimp:

- 1 pound large shrimp, peeled and deveined
- 2 tablespoons olive oil
- 1 teaspoon garlic powder
- 1 teaspoon paprika
- Salt and pepper to taste

For Salad:

- 6 cups baby spinach and kale mix
- 1 cup cherry tomatoes, halved
- 1/4 cup red onion, thinly sliced

For Light Olive Oil Dressing:

- 3 tablespoons extra virgin olive oil
- 2 tablespoons balsamic vinegar
- 1 teaspoon Dijon mustard
- 1 teaspoon honey (optional, for sweetness)
- Salt and pepper to taste

Instructions:

Grilled Shrimp:

1. In a bowl, mix olive oil, garlic powder, paprika, salt and pepper to create a marinade.

2. Add the peeled and deveined shrimp to the marinade ensuring they are well-coated.

3. Preheat the grill to medium-high heat. Thread the shrimp on skewers.

4. Grill the shrimp for about 2-3 minutes per side or until they are opaque and cooked through.

5. Once cooked remove the shrimp from the skewers and set aside.

Salad:

1. In a large salad bowl, combine the baby spinach and kale mix, halved cherry tomatoes and thinly sliced red onion.

Light Olive Oil Dressing:

1. In a small bowl or jar whisk together extra virgin olive oil, balsamic vinegar, Dijon mustard, honey (if using) salt and pepper.

2. Taste the dressing and adjust the seasoning or sweetness to your liking.

Assembling the Dish:

1. Add the grilled shrimp to the salad.

2. Drizzle the light olive oil dressing over the salad and shrimp.

3. Toss the salad gently to coat everything with the dressing.

4. Serve the Spinach and Kale Salad with Grilled Shrimp immediately.

Dinner: Baked cod with quinoa and roasted Brussels sprouts.

Ingredients:

For Baked Cod:

- 4 cod filets (about 6 oz each)
- 2 tablespoons olive oil
- 2 cloves garlic, minced
- 1 teaspoon dried thyme
- 1 teaspoon paprika
- Salt and pepper to taste
- Lemon wedges for serving

For Quinoa:

- 1 cup quinoa, rinsed
- 2 cups vegetable or chicken broth
- Salt to taste

For Roasted Brussels Sprouts:

- 1 pound Brussels sprouts, trimmed and halved
- 2 tablespoons olive oil
- Salt and pepper to taste

Instructions:

Baked Cod:

1. Preheat the oven to 400°F (200°C).
2. Place cod filets on a baking sheet lined with parchment paper.
3. In a small bowl, mix olive oil, minced garlic, dried thyme, paprika, salt and pepper.
4. Brush the cod filets with the seasoned olive oil mixture ensuring they are well-coated.
5. Bake in the preheated oven for about 12-15 minutes or until the cod easily flakes with a fork.
6. Once cooked squeeze lemon wedges over the baked cod before serving.

Quinoa:

1. In a saucepan combine quinoa and broth. Bring to a boil.
2. Reduce the heat to low, cover and simmer for about 15 minutes or until the quinoa is cooked and the liquid is absorbed.
3. Fluff the quinoa with a fork and season with salt to taste.

Roasted Brussels Sprouts:

1. Preheat the oven to 400°F (200°C).
2. Toss halved Brussels sprouts with olive oil, salt and pepper on a baking sheet.
3. Roast in the preheated oven for about 20-25 minutes or until the Brussels sprouts are golden brown and crispy on the edges.

Assembling the Dish:

1. Serve the baked cod filets over a bed of cooked quinoa.

2. Arrange the roasted Brussels sprouts on the side.

3. Garnish with additional lemon wedges if desired.

4. Enjoy this balanced and nutritious meal of Baked Cod with Quinoa and Roasted Brussels Sprouts!

Day 6:

Breakfast: Smoothie bowl with blended berries, banana and a sprinkle of hemp seeds topped with granola.

Ingredients:

- 1 cup mixed berries (strawberries, blueberries, raspberries)
- 1 ripe banana, peeled and sliced
- 1/2 cup Greek yogurt
- 1/4 cup almond milk (or any milk of your choice)
- 1 tablespoon honey (optional, for added sweetness)
- 2 tablespoons hemp seeds
- 1/2 cup granola

Instructions:

1. In a blender, combine mixed berries, sliced banana, Greek yogurt, almond milk and honey (if using).

2. Blend the ingredients until smooth and creamy. Add more almond milk if needed to achieve your desired consistency.

3. Pour the smoothie into a bowl.

4. Sprinkle hemp seeds evenly over the smoothie bowl.

5. Top the bowl with a generous amount of granola.

6. Optionally, add additional slices of fresh banana or berries for garnish.

7. Serve the Smoothie Bowl with Blended Berries, Banana, Hemp Seeds and Granola immediately.

8. Enjoy this delicious and nutrient-packed smoothie bowl!

Lunch: Vegetable and lentil curry with turmeric-infused brown rice.

Ingredients:

For Vegetable and Lentil Curry:

- 1 cup dry lentils (green or brown), rinsed
- 2 tablespoons olive oil
- 1 large onion, diced
- 3 cloves garlic, minced
- 1 tablespoon ginger, grated
- 2 carrots, peeled and sliced
- 1 bell pepper, diced
- 1 zucchini, sliced
- 1 can (14 oz) diced tomatoes
- 1 can (14 oz) coconut milk
- 2 tablespoons curry powder
- 1 teaspoon ground cumin
- 1 teaspoon ground coriander
- 1/2 teaspoon turmeric
- 1/2 teaspoon red chili flakes (optional for heat)
- Salt and pepper to taste
- Fresh cilantro, chopped (for garnish)

For Turmeric-Infused Brown Rice:

- 1 cup brown rice
- 2 cups vegetable broth
- 1 teaspoon ground turmeric
- Salt to taste

Instructions:

Vegetable and Lentil Curry:

1. In a large pot, heat olive oil over medium heat. Add diced onion and cook until softened.
2. Add minced garlic and grated ginger sauteing for another 1-2 minutes until fragrant.
3. Stir in curry powder, ground cumin, ground coriander, turmeric and red chili flakes (if using), coating the onion mixture.
4. Add sliced carrots, diced bell pepper and sliced zucchini to the pot. Cook for 5-7 minutes until the vegetables begin to soften.
5. Pour in the rinsed lentils, diced tomatoes (with their juice) and coconut milk. Season with salt and pepper.
6. Bring the curry to a simmer, then reduce the heat to low and cover. Let it cook for 25-30 minutes or until the lentils are tender and the flavors have melded.
7. Taste and adjust the seasoning if necessary.
8. Garnish the curry with chopped fresh cilantro before serving.

Turmeric-Infused Brown Rice:

1. In a saucepan, combine brown rice, vegetable broth, ground turmeric and salt.
2. Bring to a boil, then reduce the heat to low, cover and simmer for about 40-45 minutes or until the rice is tender and the liquid is absorbed.
3. Fluff the rice with a fork before serving.

Assembling the Dish:

1. Serve the Vegetable and Lentil Curry over a bed of Turmeric-Infused Brown Rice.
2. Garnish with additional fresh cilantro if desired.
3. Enjoy this wholesome and flavorful Vegetable and Lentil Curry with Turmeric-Infused Brown Rice!

Dinner: Grilled turkey or tofu burgers with a side of sweet potato wedges.

Ingredients:

For Grilled Turkey or Tofu Burgers:

- 1 pound ground turkey OR 1 package extra-firm tofu, drained and pressed
- 1/4 cup breadcrumbs (for turkey burgers)
- 1 egg (for turkey burgers)
- 2 tablespoons olive oil
- 1 teaspoon garlic powder
- 1 teaspoon onion powder
- 1 teaspoon dried thyme
- Salt and pepper to taste
- Burger buns

For Sweet Potato Wedges:

- 2 large sweet potatoes, washed and cut into wedges
- 2 tablespoons olive oil
- 1 teaspoon paprika
- 1/2 teaspoon garlic powder
- Salt and pepper to taste

Instructions:

Grilled Turkey or Tofu Burgers:

1. If making turkey burgers in a bowl, combine ground turkey, breadcrumbs, egg, olive oil, garlic powder, onion powder, dried thyme, salt and pepper. Mix until well combined. If making tofu burgers, skip the breadcrumbs and egg. Instead, crumble the pressed tofu into a bowl and mix with the other ingredients.
2. Divide the mixture into equal portions and shape them into burger patties.
3. Preheat the grill to medium-high heat.
4. Grill the turkey or tofu burgers for about 5-7 minutes per side or until fully cooked. Ensure turkey burgers reach an internal temperature of 165°F (74°C).

5. Toast the burger buns on the grill during the last minute of cooking.

6. Once cooked, assemble the burgers by placing the patties on the toasted buns. Add your favorite toppings and condiments.

Sweet Potato Wedges:

1. Preheat the oven to 425°F (220°C).

2. In a bowl, toss sweet potato wedges with olive oil, paprika, garlic powder, salt and pepper until evenly coated.

3. Spread the wedges in a single layer on a baking sheet lined with parchment paper.

4. Roast in the preheated oven for 25-30 minutes or until the sweet potato wedges are golden brown and crispy on the edges, flipping them halfway through.

Assembling the Dish:

1. Serve the Grilled Turkey or Tofu Burgers on toasted buns.

2. Serve the Sweet Potato Wedges on the side.

Day 7:

Breakfast: Chia seed pudding made with coconut milk topped with sliced mango.

Ingredients:

- 1/4 cup chia seeds
- 1 cup coconut milk (canned or from a carton)
- 1 tablespoon maple syrup or honey (optional for sweetness)
- 1/2 teaspoon vanilla extract
- 1 ripe mango, peeled and sliced

Instructions:

1. In a bowl, combine chia seeds, coconut milk, maple syrup or honey (if using) and vanilla extract.

2. Whisk the ingredients together until well combined.

3. Cover the bowl and refrigerate the chia seed mixture for at least 3-4 hours or overnight, allowing it to thicken. Stir occasionally during the first hour to prevent clumping.

4. Once the chia pudding has reached a thick pudding-like consistency give it a final stir.

5. Spoon the chia seed pudding into serving glasses or bowls.

6. Top the chia pudding with sliced mango.

7. Optionally, drizzle a bit of extra honey or maple syrup on top for added sweetness.

8. Serve the Coconut Chia Seed Pudding with Sliced Mango immediately.

9. Enjoy this delightful and nutrition breakfast!

Lunch: Mixed greens salad with grilled chicken, cherry tomatoes, cucumber and a lemon-tahini dressing.

Ingredients:

For Grilled Chicken:

- 2 boneless, skinless chicken breasts
- 2 tablespoons olive oil
- 1 teaspoon dried oregano
- Salt and pepper to taste

For Mixed Greens Salad:

- 6 cups mixed salad greens (lettuce, spinach, arugula, etc.)
- 1 cup cherry tomatoes, halved
- 1 cucumber, sliced
- 1/4 cup red onion, thinly sliced

For Lemon-Tahini Dressing:

- 3 tablespoons tahini
- 2 tablespoons olive oil
- 2 tablespoons lemon juice
- 1 clove garlic, minced

- Salt and pepper to taste

Instructions:

Grilled Chicken:

1. Preheat the grill to medium-high heat.
2. In a bowl, mix olive oil, dried oregano, salt and pepper.
3. Brush the chicken breasts with the seasoned olive oil mixture ensuring they are well-coated.
4. Grill the chicken for about 6-8 minutes per side or until cooked through. Ensure the internal temperature reaches 165°F (74°C).
5. Once cooked, let the chicken rest for a few minutes before slicing.

Mixed Greens Salad:

1. In a large salad bowl, combine mixed salad greens, halved cherry tomatoes, sliced cucumber and thinly sliced red onion.

Lemon-Tahini Dressing:

1. In a small bowl or jar, whisk together tahini, olive oil, lemon juice, minced garlic, salt, and pepper.
2. Taste the dressing and adjust the seasoning if necessary.

Assembling the Dish:

1. Arrange the grilled chicken slices on top of the mixed greens salad.
2. Drizzle the lemon-tahini dressing over the salad and chicken.
3. Toss the salad gently to coat everything with the dressing.
4. Optionally, garnish with additional lemon wedges or fresh herbs.
5. Serve the Mixed Greens Salad with Grilled Chicken and Lemon-Tahini Dressing.
6. Enjoy this light and flavorful salad with a perfect combination of greens, grilled chicken and a tangy tahini dressing!

Dinner: Quinoa-stuffed bell peppers with black beans, corn and diced tomatoes.

Ingredients:

- 4 large bell peppers, halved and seeds removed
- 1 cup quinoa, rinsed
- 2 cups vegetable broth
- 1 can (15 oz) black beans, drained and rinsed
- 1 cup corn kernels (fresh, frozen or canned)
- 1 cup diced tomatoes
- 1 teaspoon ground cumin
- 1 teaspoon chili powder
- 1/2 teaspoon smoked paprika
- Salt and pepper to taste
- 1 cup shredded cheese (cheddar, Monterey Jack or your choice)
- Fresh cilantro, chopped (for garnish)
- Lime wedges (for serving)

Instructions:

1. Preheat the oven to 375°F (190°C).
2. In a saucepan, combine quinoa and vegetable broth. Bring to a boil, then reduce heat to low, cover and simmer for about 15-20 minutes or until the quinoa is cooked and the liquid is absorbed.
3. In a large bowl, mix cooked quinoa, black beans, corn, diced tomatoes, ground cumin, chili powder, smoked paprika, salt and pepper.
4. Place the bell pepper halves in a baking dish.
5. Stuff each bell pepper half with the quinoa mixture, pressing it down slightly.
6. Sprinkle shredded cheese on top of each stuffed pepper.
7. Cover the baking dish with aluminum foil.

8. Bake in the preheated oven for 25-30 minutes or until the peppers are tender.

9. Remove the foil and bake for an additional 5-7 minutes or until the cheese is melted and bubbly.

10. Garnish with chopped fresh cilantro.

11. Serve the Quinoa-Stuffed Bell Peppers with Lime Wedges on the side.

SHOPPING LISTS

Produce:

- Leafy greens (spinach, kale, arugula)
- Citrus fruits (oranges, lemons, grapefruits)
- Berries (blueberries, strawberries, raspberries)
- Cucumbers
- Watermelon
- Avocado

Vegetables:

- Broccoli
- Cauliflower
- Celery
- Garlic
- Ginger
- Turmeric

Proteins:

- Poultry (chicken, turkey)
- Fish (salmon, trout)
- Tofu

Healthy Fats:

- Avocado
- Olive oil
- Nuts (almonds, walnuts)

Herbs and Spices:

- Basil
- Cilantro
- Dill
- Turmeric powder
- Ginger powder

Beverages:

- Herbal teas (dandelion, ginger)
- Plenty of water

Lymphatic Health Lifestyle Shopping List:

Exercise and Movement:

- Comfortable walking shoes
- Yoga mat
- Resistance bands
- Trampoline (for rebounding exercises)
- Swimwear (for swimming)

Stress Management:

- Meditation cushion or chair
- Essential oils (lavender, chamomile)
- Art supplies (canvas, paints, brushes)
- Journal or diary

General Wellness:

- Dry brush for skin brushing
- Massage oil or lotion
- Quality sleep accessories (comfortable pillows, blackout curtains)
- Nature-friendly products for outdoor activities (hiking boots, sunscreen)

LIFESTYLE TIPS FOR LYMPHATIC HEALTH

1. Keep Hydrated: Adequate water consumption is essential for lymphatic health. Maintain hydration to aid in the passage of lymphatic fluid.
2. Regular Exercise: To enhance lymphatic circulation, engage in activities that promote movement such as brisk walking, yoga or rebounding exercises.
3. Dry brushing: Incorporate dry brushing into your routine to exfoliate the skin gently and encourage lymphatic movement which promotes detoxification.
4. Deep Breathing: Engage in deep breathing exercises to improve oxygenation and lymph movement throughout the body.
5. Massage: Get regular massages, particularly ones that focus on lymphatic drainage techniques to stimulate lymphatic vessels and reduce fluid retention.
6. Elevate Your Legs: If possible, elevate your legs on a regular basis to aid lymphatic drainage, reduce edema and promote circulation.
7. Avoid Tight Clothing: Wear loose-fitting clothing to avoid constriction and allow for free lymphatic flow.
8. Maintain a healthy diet rich in fruits and vegetables, lean meats and whole grains to supply critical elements that support lymphatic function.
9. Manage Stress: Incorporate stress-reduction practices such as meditation, deep breathing or mindfulness to boost general well-being as stress has been shown to have an effect on lymphatic health.
10. Heat therapy, such as saunas or hot baths, can assist open lymphatic channels and promote detoxification. Take a sauna or a warm bath every now and again.
11. Prioritize adequate and quality sleep because the body's repair and detoxification functions are heightened during peaceful sleep.

EXERCISE AND MOVEMENT

1. Brisk walking is a simple yet efficient workout that increases lymphatic circulation and general cardiovascular health.

2. Yoga: Incorporate yoga positions that entail mild stretching and bending to improve flexibility and lymphatic drainage.

3. Bouncing on a trampoline or participating in rebounding activities helps activate the lymphatic system, making it a fun and beneficial workout.

4. Swimming: Because of the buoyancy and resistance provided by water swimming is an excellent low-impact workout that promotes lymphatic circulation.

5. Cycling: Going for a bike ride not only improves cardiovascular fitness but also promotes lymphatic drainage through rhythmic movement.

6. Incorporate resistance exercise to increase muscle, which can help with lymphatic fluid circulation and general metabolic health.

7. Pilates is a low-impact exercise that focuses on core strength and regulated movements, benefiting both the lymphatic and musculoskeletal systems.

8. Jumping rope is a dynamic and exciting sport that can increase your heart rate while also encouraging lymphatic circulation.

9. Dance: Whether at a dance studio or at home, the rhythmic and expressive movements of dance can be a pleasurable method to maintain lymphatic health.

10. Tai Chi: This ancient Chinese practice combines soft motions and deep breathing to promote relaxation and lymphatic fluid flow.

www.ingramcontent.com/pod-product-compliance
Lightning Source LLC
Chambersburg PA
CBHW070929260726
48661CB00003B/900